Rosemary Conley's
Slim to Win
Diet and Cookbook

Rosemary Conley is the UK's most successful diet and fitness expert. Her diet and fitness books, videos and DVDs have consistently topped the bestseller lists with combined sales in excess of nine million copies.

Rosemary has also presented more than 400 cookery programmes on television and has hosted several of her own TV series including *Slim to Win with Rosemary Conley*, which was first broadcast in ITV Central and Thames Valley regions in 2007, with a new series in 2008.

In 1999 Rosemary was made a Deputy Lieutenant of Leicestershire. In 2001 she was given the Freedom of the City of Leicester, and in 2004 she was awarded a CBE in the Queen's New Year Honours List for 'services to the fitness and diet industries'.

Together with her husband, Mike Rimmington, Rosemary runs four companies: Rosemary Conley Diet and Fitness Clubs, which operates an award-winning national network of almost 200 franchises running more than 2000 classes weekly; Quorn House Publishing Ltd, which publishes *Rosemary Conley Diet and Fitness* magazine; Rosemary Conley Licences Ltd; and Rosemary Conley Enterprises.

Rosemary has a daughter, Dawn, from her first marriage. Rosemary, Mike and Dawn are all committed Christians.

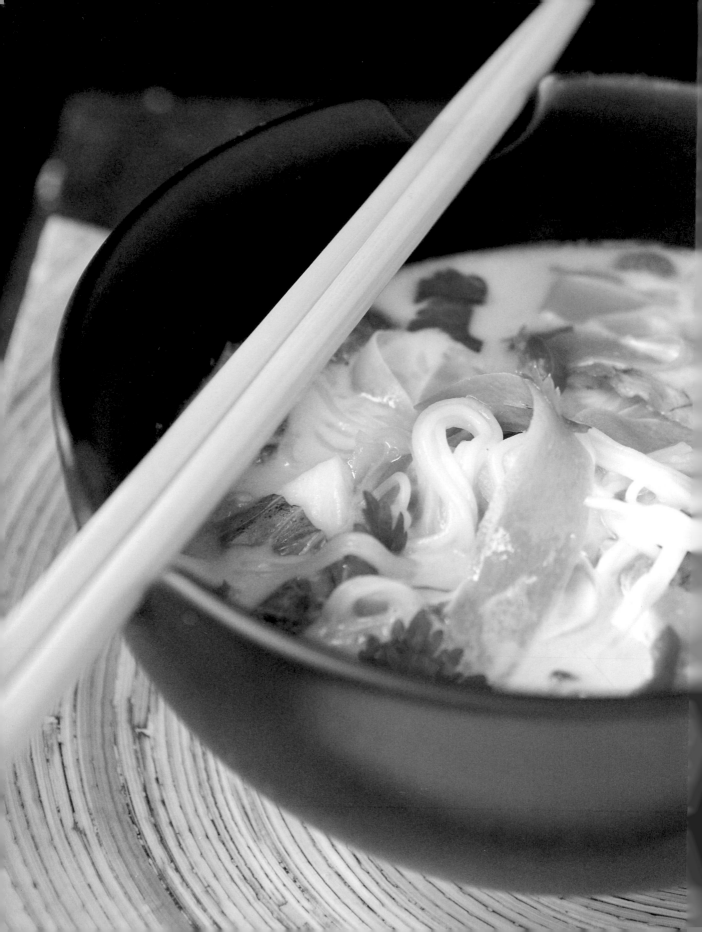

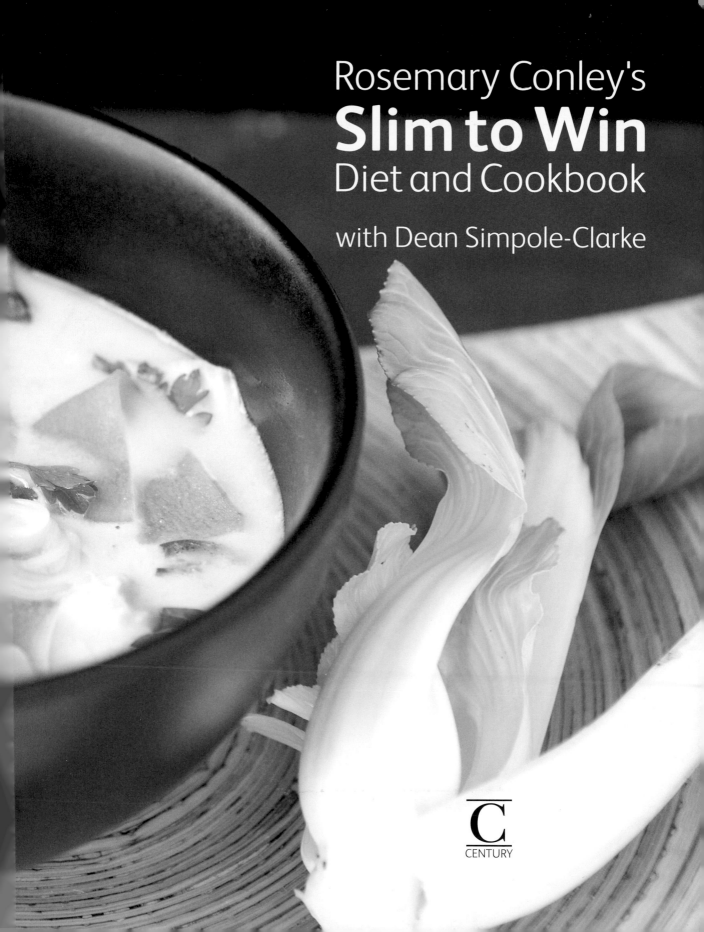

Rosemary Conley's
Slim to Win
Diet and Cookbook

with Dean Simpole-Clarke

C

CENTURY

This edition published in the United Kingdom by Century in 2010

10 9 8 7 6 5 4 3 2 1

Century
Random House UK Limited
20 Vauxhall Bridge Road, London SW1V 2SA

Addresses for companies within The Random House Group Ltd can be found at www.randomhouse.co.uk/offices.htm

The Random House UK Limited Reg. No. 954009

A CIP catalogue record for this book is available from the British Library

The Random House Group Ltd makes every effort to ensure that papers used in its books are made from trees that have been legally sourced from well-managed and credibly certified forests. Our paper procurement policy can be found at www.randomhouse.co.uk/paper.htm

ISBN 9781846053221

Food photography by Clive Doyle
Designed by Roger Walker

Printed and bound in Germany by
Firmengruppe APPL, Aprinta Druck, Wemding

Also by Rosemary Conley

Rosemary Conley's Hip and Thigh Diet

Rosemary Conley's Complete Hip and Thigh Diet

Rosemary Conley's Inch Loss Plan

Rosemary Conley's Hip and Thigh Diet Cookbook (with Patricia Bourne)

Rosemary Conley's Metabolism Booster Diet

Rosemary Conley's Whole Body Programme

Rosemary Conley's New Hip and Thigh Diet Cookbook (with Patricia Bourne)

Shape Up for Summer

Rosemary Conley's Beach Body Plan

Rosemary Conley's Flat Stomach Plan

Be Slim! Be Fit!

Rosemary Conley's Complete Flat Stomach Plan

Rosemary Conley's New Body Plan

Rosemary Conley's New Inch Loss Plan

Rosemary Conley's Low Fat Cookbook

Rosemary Conley's Red Wine Diet

Rosemary Conley's Low Fat Cookbook Two

Rosemary Conley's Eat Yourself Slim

Rosemary Conley's Step by Step Low Fat Cookbook

Rosemary Conley's Gi Jeans Diet

Rosemary Conley's Ultimate Gi Jeans Diet

Rosemary Conley's Gi Hip and Thigh Diet

Rosemary Conley's Amazing Inch Loss Plan

The diet in this book is based on sound healthy eating principles. However, it is important to check with your doctor or GP before following any weight-reducing plan. Diabetics should always follow the eating guidelines recommended by their GP or medical practitioner

Contents

Acknowledgements

This book would not have been possible without the help of my wonderful support team.

Chef Dean Simpole-Clarke has created a fabulous array of recipes, including some favourites from my *Diet & Fitness* magazine, for you to enjoy as you slim to win your figure back. Dean works closely with me in many aspects of my work – my books, my magazine and on television, including my *Slim to Win* series. Thank you, Dean.

Special thanks must go to my editor, Jan Bowmer, without whom my books would not make it to the general public! Jan has worked with me for almost 20 years, and her understanding of my philosophy, and how I aim for it to be conveyed to the reader, is remarkable. Her amazing, computer-like memory ensures fastidious attention to detail. Jan has worked incredibly hard to ensure that this book will be easy for you to use and practical for you to follow. I am so grateful to you, Jan, for all your talent and immense hard work, as always. Thank you. You are a star!

In any cookbook, photographs are crucial. Food photographer Clive Doyle has done a superb job in capturing the colour and textures of the food to tempt your taste buds. Clive is a joy to work with, and he and Dean make a great team. Thank you, Clive.

My super secretary, Anja Zeman, did a sterling job in calculating the fat and calorie content of each recipe throughout this book. Thank you for being such a willing and able calculator and right-hand-woman! Also, many thanks to my daughter, Dawn, who helped and supported me in the creation of the diet and meal selections for this book as well as for my Gi Hip and Thigh Diet, on which this Slim to Win diet is based. You are a real inspiration and I value you so much. Thanks are also due to the rest of the team at Quorn House, our head office, for the various tasks you were asked to complete to help this book meet its deadline.

Designer Roger Walker has done a brilliant job in making this book look attractive and easy to use. Thank you for all your hard work, Roger.

Thanks also to Hannah Black, and the rest of the team at Century, for commissioning this book in the first place.

Last, but by no means least, I want to thank ITV Central, for commissioning the *Slim to Win with Rosemary Conley* series, and my television dieters who have been a total delight to work with. I hope you enjoy lifetime success in your fitter and slimmer bodies! Thank you all so much.

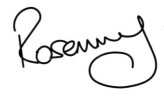

Useful information

Body weight conversions

Pound (lb)	Stone (st)	Kilogram (kg)
1		0.5
2		1
3		1.4
4		1.8
5		2.3
6		2.7
7	½	3.2
8		3.6
9		4.1
10		4.5
11		5
12		5.4
13		5.9
14	1	6.3
28	2	12.7

Abbreviations and symbols used

lb	pound
g	gram
kg	kilogram
st	stone
ml	millilitre
in	inch
foot	ft
mm	millimetre
cm	centimetre
kcal	calorie
✓	suitable for vegetarians
❄	suitable for home freezing

Spoon measures

1 teaspoon = 5ml	
1 tablespoon = 15ml	

Visit www.rosemaryconley.com for more diet and fitness advice.

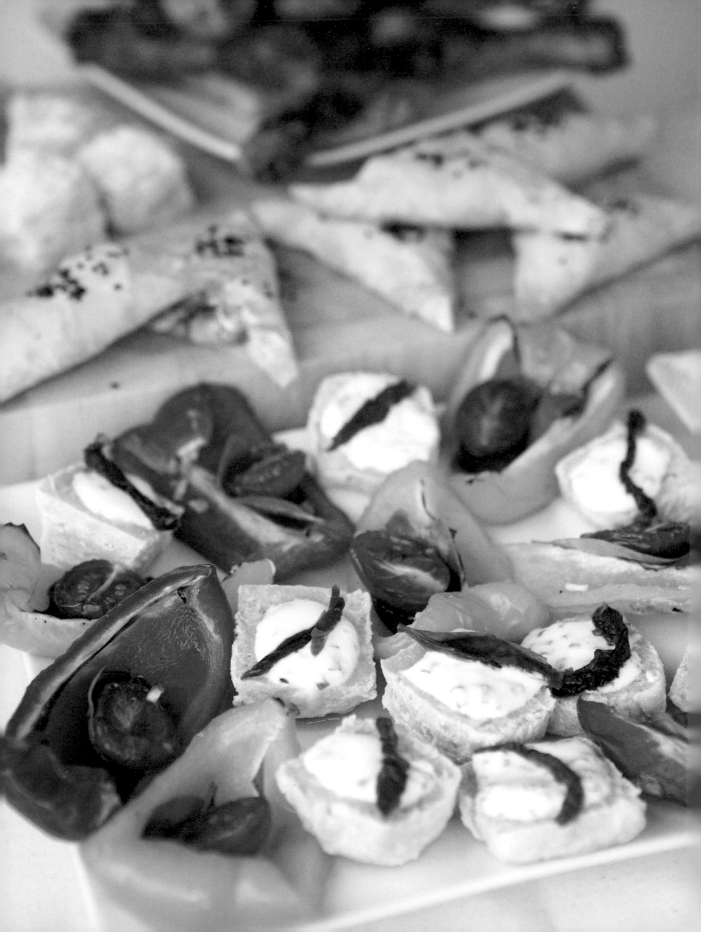

Your life-changing journey starts here

Anyone who slims down and regains their youthful figure is a winner. There is no price you can place on looking – and feeling – ten years younger, easing your aching joints and having energy to spare at the end of the day.

Based on the priciples of my best-selling *Gi Hip and Thigh Diet* (Arrow), this book accompanies my second television series of *Slim to Win with Rosemary Conley* on ITV Central. The series follows seven overweight men and women on a life-changing journey to re-educate their eating habits and adopt a more active lifestyle. If it's not aired in your area, you can log on to www.itvlocal. com or our own website www.rosemaryconley.com and watch each episode as it unfolds.

However, this book is about helping YOU. I have included the same diet principles, activity advice and motivational tips that my television slimmers followed and, although I didn't have their final results before this book went to print, after just two months on the diet, this is the progress they had made:

Alan Graves lost 1st 9lb

Lauren Hewitt lost 8lb

Debra Gaskin lost 1st 6lb

Vicky Argyle lost 1st 8lb

Roweena Kaur lost 1st 8lb

Allyson Wicklen lost 1st 7lb

Neil Wicklen (Allyson's father) lost 2st 9lb

It worked for them and it can work for you. I will show you how to make some common-sense choices about the food you eat – what to buy and how to cook it – and what activity to do.

For more than 35 years I've been helping people to get slim, and during that exciting and enjoyable career I've had the privilege of working with some of the UK's top experts in the fields of nutrition (Professor Andrew Prentice and Dr Susan Jebb), exercise physiology (Professor Kevin Sykes), psychology (Professor Raj Persaud), general medicine (Dr Hilary Jones), as well as exercise and weight management (Mary Morris Msc) and cookery (chef Dean Simpole-Clarke).

I have learned so much from these people and incorporated their very best advice into many of my diet and fitness programmes – in my books, videos and DVDs, my *Diet & Fitness* magazine, Rosemary Conley Diet and Fitness Clubs and our online slimming club, www.rosemaryconleyonline.com, and now in my *Slim to Win* series for ITV. Indeed, most of these experts have appeared in the programme.

This diet and cookbook gives you the tools you need to change your lifestyle for the better by losing your unwanted weight and getting fitter, just as my Slim to Win dieters did. It is easier than you think, but only *you* can decide that you want to be a winner. No one can do it for you, but once you start to see results you'll be so encouraged that you will transform your body faster than you ever thought possible.

Chef Dean Simpole-Clarke has provided a wonderful array of dishes suitable for all the family, including some special recipes he created for my Slim to Win dieters, who featured in the series. Those recipes are prefixed with the dieter's name. The calorie and fat content is clearly shown with every recipe throughout the book.

I've included a strict Fat Attack Fortnight Diet to get you started on your weight-loss journey. The initial short, sharp, concerted effort will pay dividends by enabling you to lose around 7lb in the first two weeks! Then, from week three you can enjoy alcohol, puddings and treats, depending on your personal calorie allowance, which you can calculate by referring to the tables on pages 278–9. I've given some additional menus so you can continue your weight-loss programme as well as advice on how to become more active, how to cook the low fat way, plus some motivational tips. In addition, there are lots of extra recipes to stimulate your taste buds, whether you are dieting or entertaining friends. As all the calories are stated per serving throughout, it's easy to incorporate these into your daily calorie allowance.

Use the charts at the back of the book to monitor your weight and inch loss progress and be aware that you'll not only be transforming the outside appearance of your body but the inside, too!

Perfect portion control

Overestimating portion sizes is the biggest single reason why dieters don't lose weight as fast as they think they deserve to.

Rosemary Conley Portion Pots, which come in four different sizes and colour, offer a simple solution for measuring your servings of staple foods such as rice, pasta, cereals, baked beans, chopped foods – and even wine. Once you get into the habit of using them, you'll speed up your weight loss like a dream. To order a set, visit www.rosemaryconley.com or call 0870 050 7727. They cost just £4.99 plus p&p or get a set free when you join your local Rosemary Conley Diet and Fitness Club.

I have included the appropriate portion pot colour in the diet and menu plans on pages 20–35 to help you measure your servings with greater accuracy and ease, but in case you do not yet own a set I have also given the equivalent metric weight equivalents.

How to be a weight-loss winner

The key to losing weight successfully is to eat fewer calories than your body uses up in energy, so that it calls on its fat stores to make up the difference. At the same time, if you burn extra calories by being more active you will dramatically speed up your weight-loss progress.

The good news is that, by making informed choices about the type of foods you eat, you can eat well and still lose weight safely and effectively without necessarily reducing the quantity of food you actually consume. The best way to do this is to follow a healthy, low-fat diet. If, at the same time, you increase your activity levels you will lose weight even faster. It's a win-win situation.

Cut back on calories and fat

Fat (oil, butter, margarine, etc) provides twice as many calories, gram for gram, as found in carbohydrate (rice, pasta, potatoes, bread and cereal) or protein (meat, fish, eggs, cheese and milk), so the obvious first step is to cut down on fat. By selecting foods with a maximum of 5% fat (5 grams of fat per 100 grams of food), you will reduce your calorie intake quite significantly without having to eat less food.

Fill up on healthy, low-Gi foods

Gi stands for glycaemic index, which rates foods on the speed at which they are digested and absorbed into the bloodstream. Foods with a low Gi are slowly digested, which helps us to feel fuller for longer. And this, of course, is a great aid when we are trying to lose weight. Studies show that a low-Gi eating plan can also help to reduce our risk of developing diabetes or heart disease.

Eating low-Gi foods prevents those sudden food cravings that are the main reason dieters fail to lose weight. In a moment of hunger they reach for that sugary or high-fat snack which can ruin the most effective of diets.

Follow a balanced, healthy eating plan

A low-Gi diet is based around fibre-rich foods and includes lots of fresh fruit and vegetables and generous helpings of beans and pulses.

When following my Slim to Win diet plan, be aware that not EVERY food you eat needs to be low Gi. The aim is to eat a balanced, healthy diet that contains a high proportion of low- or medium-Gi foods and to choose healthy, low-fat options. Adding just one low-Gi food to your meal will reduce its Gi rating.

Ten tips for successful slimming

1 **Eat three meals a day** and a small Power Snack mid-morning and mid-afternoon.

2 **Watch your portion sizes** Use my Portion Pots opposite for measuring out basic foods to make sure you are eating the correct amount.

3 **Cook without fat** With non-stick pans it is really simple to prepare foods without adding fat or oil. It doesn't take long to change your taste buds, and switching to low-fat eating is the quickest way to cut

down on hundreds of calories and loads of fat grams.

4 **Plan ahead** Make a list of foods you need to buy each week and stick to it. Don't be seduced by special offers at the supermarket, because you might be tempted to eat up extra foods to avoid throwing them away once their best-before date has expired.

5 **Eat the low-Gi way** Eating low-Gi foods will help you feel fuller for longer and so avoid temptation.

6 **Get moving!** Being more active in your everyday life will speed up your weight-loss progress, and doing any form of exercise that makes you breathe more deeply, such as brisk walking, jogging or an aerobics class, will burn fat!

7 **Wear a pedometer** It's a great motivational tool and will make you more aware of your activity levels. Aim to do 10,000 steps a day and, if you can't avoid having a sedentary day occasionally, do extra steps the next day!

8 **Mix with positive people** At a Rosemary Conley Diet and Fitness Club you'll be made to feel welcome and get support and encouragement from qualified instructors as well as mix with like-minded folk who want to lose weight, just like you. Visit our website: www.rosemaryconley.com to find details of classes near you. Or, join our internet-based diet and fitness club: rosemaryconleyonline.

9 **Avoid snacking between meals** Eating high-fat, sugary snacks between meals is one of the main reasons why people gain weight. Stop the habit and you'll transform your rate of weight loss – and your figure.

10 **Celebrate your success** by rewarding yourself every time you lose a stone or reach a new, significant milestone, such as fitting into a smaller dress size or having to take in your belt a notch.

Get the family on side

Only *you* can decide whether you want to lose weight, eat healthily and exercise regularly. But you're much more likely to succeed if other family members join in and make some lifestyle changes too.

Changing habits

Parents are the best role models for children and should aim to lay down the foundations of healthy eating so that good habits are learnt early on. That doesn't mean you can't ever, as a family, go to McDonald's or KFC, or eat chocolate or popcorn. You can – occasionally.

The key is to instil some structure into the family's eating habits – e.g. three meals a day and no snacking on high-fat foods in between. Making simple changes in the way you shop and cook can have a dramatic effect. I know women who've done this without telling their husbands or partners. The latter have assumed they're eating exactly the same food as before and yet ended up losing a stone or so!

So start slowly, making only a few subtle changes initially.

Shopping

Swap high-fat, high-calorie dressings and sauces for low-fat ones. Avoid buying biscuits if you can and buy more fruit instead. Most children enjoy eating bananas, and satsumas are delicious and easy to peel. Kiwi fruits are also fun to eat if you remove their tops and eat with a teaspoon. If the family insist on some savoury snacks, look out for the very low-fat varieties.

Choose lean cuts of meat, and aim to buy more chicken and fish and cut down on the amount of red meat. Experiment with different kinds of vegetables.

Preparing food

Cooking without adding oil, lard or butter will significantly reduce the calories and fat in your meals. Only very young children (under two years) need to have some extra fat in their diet and this can be achieved by giving them cheese and full-fat milk.

I never add oil, fat or butter to food when cooking, even if the instructions on a packet or jar say I should. When I make a cottage pie or spaghetti bolognese, I dry-fry the minced beef and then drain it through a colander before adding other ingredients. This saves lots of unwanted fat without spoiling the flavour or texture.

Try dry-roasting sweet potatoes and parsnips for a change. Just par-boil them with a vegetable stock cube for five minutes and then place on a baking tray at the top of a hot oven for 40 minutes, or until they go golden brown.

When making sandwiches, rather than using butter or a low-fat spread (most are still very high in fat), use a low-fat sauce or dressing instead. Try Branston pickle, mustard, tomato ketchup or low-fat salad dressings, and spread straight on to bread before adding your choice of filling.

Likewise, don't add fat when serving food and you'll avoid eating loads of unnecessary calories. So mash your potatoes with yogurt or semi-skimmed milk instead of butter or spread. If you've cooked vegetables in water with a vegetable stock cube, you'll find there's no need to add butter and they'll taste just as good.

Use low-fat Greek-style yogurt instead of double cream or crème fraîche in desserts. Crème fraîche is still quite high in fat, whereas Greek-style yogurt can give you the creamy flavour you crave while saving lots of calories.

Treats

An essential part of family life is spending quality time together, doing things you all enjoy, and having fun. Occasionally this may involve eating some not-quite-so-healthy foods and these will do no harm if eaten in moderation.

One family I know has a 'family night' each Friday. They take turns at choosing a favourite activity (watching TV or a DVD, or playing a game) and what to eat, and everyone else has to join in without moaning! It works. It gives the children permission to indulge without any feelings of guilt – and that's healthy! You are much more likely to get the family's co-operation in creating a healthier lifestyle if there's a bit of give-and-take.

Activity

It's also important to find time for family activities such as swimming, cycling, walking, kicking a ball around, tennis, badminton, horse-riding, ice skating, or roller skating. When was the last time you all took a walk together in the local park? Try it and see how enjoyable it is.

Winning tactics

Yes, it will take a bit of effort and yes, you may come up against a bit of resistance at first, but if you handle it carefully and thoughtfully, you should be able to win your family over. Try to use gentle persuasion rather than bullying tactics. Or don't tell them at all. Just make the changes to the way you shop, cook and serve your food and maybe no one will even notice!

Alcohol – yes or no?

Drinking too much alcohol is another reason why many people find it difficult to lose weight. As alcohol doesn't satisfy our appetite in the same way as food, we like to think that it doesn't count – but I'm afraid it certainly does!

It's easy to underestimate how much we are drinking and we often forget to take account of the extra calories. On top of that, alcohol weakens our willpower, makes us feel hungry and increases our desire for fatty food.

However, it's been proven that a glass of wine a day can actually be good for us. The problem arises when we exceed that quantity.

On my Slim to Win Diet, once you've completed the Fat Attack Fortnight, you are allowed one (125ml) glass of wine every single day. If you want, you can save a few days' worth for a special occasion so you can relax and have a good time without it affecting your weight-loss progress! It's important to understand how the body deals with alcohol, though, because it is processed in a very different way from food.

During normal digestion of food, the body uses protein and carbohydrate as easy-to-burn fuel for energy. It is only when these supplies have run out that it turns to fat for its energy supplies. However, alcohol is a toxin and, as such, the body works hard to eliminate it as soon as possible. Consequently, the calories from alcohol go to the head of the queue and are burned off in preference to those from food. The problems really begin when we drink a lot of alcohol and start fancying something fatty, such as a curry perhaps? The alcohol is burned off quickly, which means the fat from the curry goes straight into storage. In this instance, the so-called 'beer belly' is from the curry, not the beer!

Remember to stay within the recommended limits – 14 units of alcohol a week for women and 21 for men. With today's generous wine measures and the varying strengths of beer and lager, it's not surprising that we often drink more than we realise. But to lose weight, it's important to count the calories from alcohol into our daily allowance or we won't see the results we're hoping for on the scales.

To help put alcohol consumption into perspective, remember that if you were to drink a whole bottle of wine you'd have to walk seven miles to burn off the calories!

Get moving – why exercise is a must

Right from the start of their slimming campaign, my Slim to Win dieters found that the key to their success was to get more active.

People who make exercise a habit often tell us how much better they look and feel, how they've never been in better shape and that they've 'found' muscles they didn't know existed. Their skin has usually taken on a special glow, radiating good health, and their hair and nails are likely to be in great condition. Overall, they have more energy for life.

So, if you want to speed up your weight loss, and look – and feel – your best, you must step up the amount of exercise you do. Choose something you enjoy so you keep it up. You'll not only see results faster but your body and skin will shrink, your body shape will improve and you'll achieve the figure you've always dreamed of!

Turn yourself into a fat-burner

Aerobic means 'with oxygen' and aerobic exercise is any activity that causes us to breathe more deeply, such as walking, jogging, cycling and, of course, working out at an aerobics class or to a fitness DVD. It's great for improving general health and fitness and the good news for slimmers is that it also burns body fat.

The heart is a muscle and, if we don't exercise it, it will become weaker. The sensation of your heart beating faster when you exert yourself – which can happen from as normal an activity as going up stairs – shows that you are stimulating the heart muscle and, in turn, making it stronger. Also, when the heart beats faster, you'll need more air coming into the lungs, so they work harder too. Finally, as the heart pumps out more blood, the circulatory system (made up of an amazing network of arteries and veins) becomes more efficient at pumping blood and oxygen to every inch of the body, right to the surface of the skin.

When we do aerobic exercise we, in effect, 'turn up the gas' and burn extra calories. Even more importantly, regular aerobic exercise causes the body to become a more efficient fat burner in everyday life – all the time. Imagine converting the engine in your car from a 1.6 litre to a 2.8 litre one – it will use more fuel!

Improve your muscle tone and body shape

Good muscle tone will give you a beautifully toned shape and good body strength to cope with everyday living. You've heard the saying 'use it or lose it'. Well, if we don't use our muscles regularly they will become smaller and weaker. As we get older our muscles naturally reduce in size and our bodies lay down more fat as our metabolic rate slows down.

When we exercise an individual muscle, that muscle becomes leaner, firmer and stronger.

Within all our muscles are what are called little 'powerhouses' (mitochondria) that multiply in number when that muscle is stimulated through exercise to cope with the extra demand, even more so if we add resistance in the form of weights, a resistance band, or by using our own body weight. These 'powerhouses' are the physical point at which fat is burned off in the body. Therefore, if you have strong, well-exercised muscles that contain loads of mitochondria, you'll be burning body fat more efficiently, resulting in a higher metabolism and an ability to lose weight more easily.

Strength and toning activities include Pilates, a multi-gym workout, free weights as well as gentler but nevertheless very effective body-conditioning exercises.

Be flexible

Whether we are reaching into a high cupboard, putting on our seat belt or zipping up the back of a dress, it's important for our bodies to be flexible. Flexibility is incorporated in many forms of exercise. At the beginning and the end of your aerobics or toning session, you should stretch your muscles to help prevent injury during the exercise and avoid aching muscles later. It also encourages greater flexibility in the joints and more elasticity in the muscles.

Get stronger bones

As we age our bones lose strength but we can slow down that process considerably by doing the right kind of exercise. Swimming, for example, is a great cardiovascular exercise that works the heart and lungs really well but has little effect on the bones.

Walking regularly has been proven to keep the thigh and hip bones relatively strong, but to strengthen the bones in the upper body you need to add some exercises that really load the bones of the wrists, arms and the shoulder area. At the same time if you eat a diet high in calcium you will be doing the very best for your bones.

Keep your joints mobile

The more active you are, the better your joint health will be. Too sedentary a lifestyle can lead to pain and stiffness in the joints. If you have a condition such as arthritis, it is best to keep moving on a regular basis. Doing some stretching exercises will ensure that you keep a good range of movement in the joint.

The best exercise for weight loss

Quite simply, if you want to speed up your weight loss your exercise should make you a bit hot and sweaty and a little out of breath and you need to exercise for 30 minutes five times a week. This doesn't have to be done in one session – three sessions of 10 minutes in a day will still be effective. If you watch your calorie intake and combine your aerobic activity with some body conditioning work to strengthen and tone the muscles, ideally using a resistance band or weights, for 10 minutes or so on three days a week, you will soon be the proud owner of a fit, trim, shapely and healthy body, one that HELPS you to stay slim because it's an efficient fat burner.

FITNESS FACTS

- Many people could increase their fitness by just adding a little more activity to their daily routine.

- We are ten times more likely to continue with a fitness programme if we do something we enjoy, so take up an energetic pastime that you love.

- To improve and maintain your fitness and help weight management, you should take part in some form of physical activity for 30 minutes five times a week.

- Stair climbing is a good exercise, so use the stairs in preference to the lift or escalator whenever possible. If you avoid climbing stairs, you are missing an opportunity to get fit and tone your backside!

- Brisk walking over a distance of at least one mile per day is an excellent form of aerobic exercise.

- Use your spare time fruitfully. Look upon your housework, lawn-mowing, dog walking and DIY as workouts – and do more!

20 ways to speed up your weight loss

When you're well on the way to reaching your weight-loss goal, it can be frustrating when you're trying so hard to lose those last few pounds but find that progress is slow. Here's how to speed things along.

1 Cut back on your portions of meat or chicken and increase your portions of vegetables. This will help to fill you up on fewer calories.

2 Stop guessing at portion sizes. Always measure out your portions (use my Portion Pots, if you have a set) of rice, pasta, cereal – and wine!

3 Drink plenty of water or reduced-calorie drinks so you stay hydrated. Sometimes when we feel peckish, it's because we're thirsty.

4 Always have a glass of water or a low-calorie drink before and during meals. It will help you to feel full more quickly.

5 Never leave items at the bottom of your stairs to take up later. Each trip upstairs will help you to burn extra calories.

6 Use your exercise time fruitfully: make that phone call to your friend on your mobile while you're taking a walk; walk rather than drive to the postbox; try walking all or most of your way to work.

7 Walk instead of taking the car when you can. If you can't manage it every day, then aim to do it at least three times a week. If you take the dog for a walk each day, aim to walk faster and further.

8 Aim to play a sport once a week. Whether it's tennis, squash, badminton or football or horse-riding, plan to do it with a friend and turn it into a social event.

9 Use a home exercise machine while watching your favourite TV programme instead of flopping out on the sofa.

10 Avoid adding olive oil – or any oil for that matter – to your food. It only adds loads of unnecessary calories and deposits fat on your body.

11 When dry-frying mince, drain away all the fat before adding the other ingredients.

12 Avoid all high-fat snacking between meals.

13 Keep a strict eye on your calorie intake and stick to your daily allowance.

14 When dining out, choose wisely and avoid dishes cooked in or with fat, such as chips, pies, cakes, deep-fried fish or chicken.

15 In restaurants, ask for food to be served without added oil or butter.

16 Drink alcohol in moderation only. Too much will weaken your willpower and give you a bigger appetite.

17 Increase the amount of activity you do by incorporating it into your everyday life. Use the stairs rather than the lift. Stand more and sit less. Walk around while the TV commercials are on.

18 Plan each day's menu ahead – and stick to it.

19 If you find it difficult to give up your favourite food, find a low-fat alternative. So if you can't live without chocolate, look for a low-fat chocolate dessert or drink, and count the calories into your daily total.

20 Remember this golden rule: if you're not losing weight, you're eating too many calories and not exercising enough. Correct these and I promise you'll start to lose weight at a steady rate again. Honestly – it works!

Slim to Win Diet

Research has shown that you are much more likely to succeed on a weight-loss programme if you see a significant weight loss early on. This is why my Slim to Win Diet offers a fairly strict eating plan for the first two weeks, followed by a more generous calorie allowance from week three onwards. In trials, we found that dieters lost, on average, a staggering 7.25lb in the first 14 days and it wasn't unusual for them to lose a stone – or more in some cases – in the first month. For instance, *Slim to Win* dieter Neil Wicklen lost an incredible 1st 9lb in the first four weeks!

What to do

For the first two weeks, follow the Fat Attack Fortnight Diet of 1200 calories a day. During these two weeks you are allowed three main meals a day and two small power snacks. You can either use the 14-day eating plan on pages 20–27 or choose your menus from the suggestions on pages 27–37. For convenience, all the meals within each category are interchangeable, so select your favourites and repeat them as often as you want.

From week three, in addition to the above meals, you can enjoy a daily treat, an alcoholic drink and a pudding if your calorie allowance permits. Use the charts on pages 278–279 to find out your personal daily calorie allowance according to your age, gender and current weight so you can design your own eating plan, choosing from the menus and recipes in this book.

Remember, you can speed up your rate of weight loss by introducing more activity or formal exercise into your daily life. *Aerobic* exercise burns fat while *toning* exercises make your muscles stronger and shapelier. To maximise your weight loss and improve your overall shape, aim to do a selection of both types several times a week, even if it's only for ten minutes at a time.

Diet notes

- Choose foods with 5% or less fat content unless otherwise stated in the diet plan.
- 'Salad' includes all salad leaves, cress, tomatoes and raw vegetables such as cucumber, peppers, carrots, onion, mushrooms, celery and courgettes, and may be served with 1 teaspoon fat-free, low-calorie dressing.
- 'Unlimited vegetables' means any vegetables, excluding potatoes, cooked and served without fat.
- '1 piece fresh fruit' means 1 medium-sized apple, orange or pear, etc., or 115g fruit such as grapes and strawberries.
- You can repeat any of the menu options as you wish to suit your taste, but aim to incorporate at least five portions a day of fruit and/or vegetables in your selections.
- Drink at least five large glasses of water a day. You can also drink unlimited tea and coffee, using milk from your allowance, and low-calorie soft drinks.
- You may take a multi-vitamin supplement each day if you wish.
- ☑ means suitable for vegetarians or vegetarian option is available.

Daily allowance

	CALORIES
450ml/¾ pint skimmed or semi-skimmed milk	200
1 Breakfast	200
1 Lunch	300
1 Dinner	400
2 Power Snacks	100
Total	1200

Remember, all meals are interchangeable within each category, e.g. you can swap or repeat any lunch suggestion for another lunch you prefer.

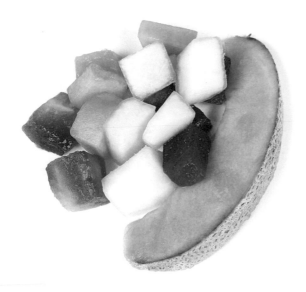

The Fat Attack Fortnight Diet

DAY 1

Breakfast ✓
½ melon filled with 1 red portion pot/115g raspberries, plus 1 low-fat fruit yogurt (max. 100 kcal and 5% fat)

Mid-morning Power Snack
2 satsumas

Lunch ✓
2 slices wholegrain bread spread with mustard or pickle, made into an open sandwich with 50g wafer-thin ham, chicken, turkey or low-fat cottage cheese, plus a small salad

Mid-afternoon Power Snack
Vegetable crudités: ½ carrot, ¼ red pepper, ¼ green pepper, 1 stick celery, 1 × 5cm piece cucumber and 5 cherry tomatoes

Dinner
Pan-Fried Liver with Leek Mash (see recipe page 180) served with unlimited vegetables (excluding potatoes),

DAY 2

Breakfast ☑
1 Weetabix served with 100g canned peaches in natural juice, 100g low-fat natural yogurt and 1 teaspoon brown sugar

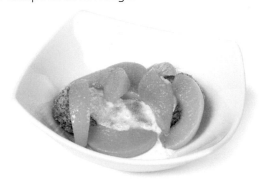

Mid-morning Power Snack
100g pomegranate seeds

Lunch
50g cooked or smoked salmon, mackerel or trout served with 1 teaspoon horseradish sauce and a large salad tossed in oil-free dressing

Mid-afternoon Power Snack
2 kiwi fruit

Dinner
1 × 150g chicken breast (no skin) chopped and dry-fried until almost cooked. Add ½ pack stir-fry vegetables and unlimited beansprouts. When hot, add soy sauce and 1 tablespoon sweet chilli sauce

Power snacks
1 × 90g Tesco Fresh Apple and Grape Snack Pack

DAY 3

Breakfast
2 grilled turkey rashers served with 1 slice wholegrain bread, toasted, plus 1 small can (approx. 200g) tomatoes, boiled until reduced

Mid-morning Power Snack
5 heaped tablespoons blueberries

Lunch ☑
1 × 400g can lentil or vegetable soup (max. 5% fat and 200 kcal) served with 1 slice wholegrain bread, toasted

Mid-afternoon Power Snack
Crudités with dip: 1 blue portion pot/75g tomato salsa, plus 5cm cucumber, 1 celery stick and ¼ yellow pepper, all cut into sticks

Dinner ☑
Mushroom and Spinach Pasta Bake (see recipe page 120) served with green salad

DAY 4

Breakfast ☑
1 red portion pot/50g bran flakes or Sultana Bran served with milk from allowance and 1 teaspoon sugar

Mid-morning Power Snack
1 yellow portion pot/70g blueberries topped with 2 teaspoons Total 0% fat Greek yogurt

Lunch ☑
1 × 150g oven-baked sweet potato topped with Carbonara, Chicken Korma or Fruity Coleslaw (see recipes pages 170–172), plus 1 piece fresh fruit (excluding bananas)

Mid-afternoon Power Snack
2 kiwi fruit

Dinner ☑
Quorn and Mushroom Stuffed Red Onions (see recipe page 151) served with 150g boiled new potatoes (with skins) and a salad

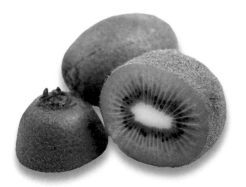

DAY 5

Breakfast ☑
1 slice wholegrain bread, toasted, spread with 1 teaspoon jam, marmalade or honey, plus 1 whole fresh grapefruit

Mid-morning Power Snack
12 seedless grapes

Lunch
2 slices wholegrain bread, spread with low-calorie salad cream and made into open sandwiches, topped with 50g wafer-thin ham, turkey, beef or smoked salmon plus a small mixed salad

Mid-afternoon Power Snack
100g pomegranate seeds

Dinner
Lamb and Pepper Hotpot (see recipe page 134) served with green vegetables

DAY 6

Breakfast
Blueberry crunch: 40g cornflakes, topped with 10g fresh blueberries, 2 tablespoons low-fat natural yogurt and 2 teaspoons maple syrup

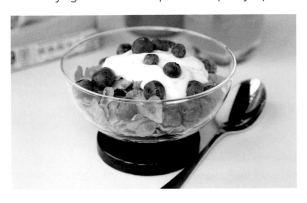

Mid-morning Power Snack
1 apple or pear

Lunch ☑
Quick two bean salad: toss 100g each drained canned kidney beans and chickpeas, 1 sliced spring onion, 2 quartered cherry tomatoes, 1 celery stick, chopped red pepper and parsley in oil-free dressing; serve with 1 wholegrain crispbread spread with 1 tablespoon half-fat cottage cheese

Mid-afternoon Power Snack
1 apple or pear

Dinner
150g white fish, steamed, served with 115g boiled new potatoes (with skins) and unlimited green vegetables

DAY 7

Breakfast ☑
1 red portion pot/60g All-Bran served with milk from allowance and 1 teaspoon sugar

Mid-morning Power Snack
2 satsumas

Lunch ☑
1 small low-fat pizza (max. 230 kcal and 5% fat) served with a large mixed salad tossed in oil-free dressing

Mid-afternoon Power Snack
Crudités with dip: 1 blue portion pot/75g tomato salsa, plus 5cm cucumber, 1 celery stick and ¼ yellow pepper, all cut into sticks

Dinner ☑
Veggie Cottage Pie (see recipe page 211) served with green vegetables or salad

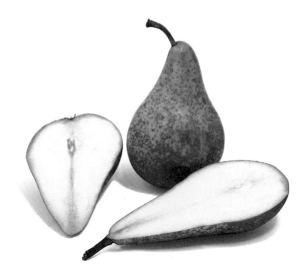

DAY 8

Breakfast ☑
1 Weetabix served with 100g canned peaches in natural juice, 100g low-fat natural yogurt and 1 teaspoon brown sugar

Mid-morning Power Snack
1 cereal bowl of mixed salad with oil-free dressing

Lunch ☑
1 × 400g can any soup (max. 5 % fat and 200 kcal) served with 1 slice toasted wholegrain bread

Mid-afternoon Power Snack
2 kiwi fruit

Dinner
Chilli Con Carne (see recipe page 139) served with a green salad

DAY 9

Breakfast
200g fresh fruit salad plus 100g low-fat yogurt (max. 5 % fat) and 1 tablespoon muesli

Mid-morning Power Snack
12 seedless grapes

Lunch ☑
2 slices wholegrain bread, toasted, topped with 1 yellow portion pot/115g baked beans

Mid-afternoon Power Snack
10 sweet silverskin pickled onions plus 10 cherry tomatoes

Dinner ☑
3 low-fat pork sausages or Quorn sausages (max. 5 % fat), grilled, served with 115g mashed sweet potatoes, unlimited green vegetables and gravy

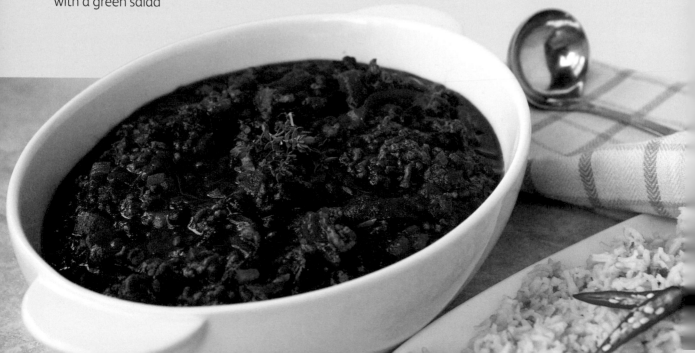

DAY 10

Breakfast
2 grilled turkey rashers served with ½ slice wholegrain bread, toasted, plus 50g baked beans

Mid-morning Power Snack
2 satsumas

Lunch ☑
Any Tasty Toast Topper (see recipes pages 168–169) plus salad and 1 piece fresh fruit (excluding bananas)

Mid-afternoon Power Snack
Tomato and basil salad: 2 tomatoes, sliced and mixed with 5 fresh basil leaves and ¼ red onion, finely chopped

Dinner ☑
Fresh Tuna with Tomato and Radish Salsa (see recipe page 184) served with 1 blue portion pot/55g (uncooked weight) or 1 red portion pot/144g (cooked weight) boiled basmati rice

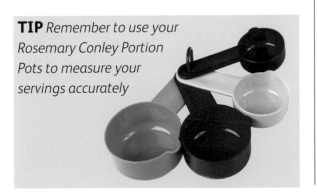

TIP *Remember to use your Rosemary Conley Portion Pots to measure your servings accurately*

DAY 11

Breakfast
1 poached or dry-fried egg served with 1 grilled low-fat sausage, 2 grilled tomatoes and 100g grilled mushrooms

Mid-morning Power Snack
2 kiwi fruit

Lunch
1 wholegrain or wholemeal tortilla wrap (max. 200 kcal) spread with 1 teaspoon sweet chilli sauce and filled with mixed salad leaves and 50g cooked chicken breast (no skin)

Mid-afternoon Power Snack
12 seedless grapes

Dinner ☑
Quorn Lasagne Verde (see recipe page 128) plus a mixed leaf salad tossed in oil-free dressing; 1 satsuma

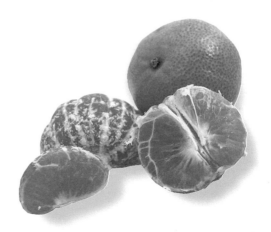

DAY 12

Breakfast ☑

1 slice wholegrain bread, toasted, topped with 100g baked beans, plus 1 whole fresh grapefruit

Mid-morning Power Snack

2 satsumas

Lunch ☑

1 × 150g oven-baked sweet potato topped with any Jacket Potato Filler (see recipes pages 170–172), plus 1 piece fresh fruit (excluding bananas)

Mid-afternoon Power Snack

5 mini low-fat breadsticks plus 1 tablespoon Total 0% fat Greek yogurt mixed with chopped chives

Dinner

Fruity Turkey Stir-Fry (see recipe page 88) served with 1 blue portion pot/55g (dry weight) or 1 red portion pot/144g (cooked weight) boiled basmati rice

DAY 13

Breakfast ☑

1 pot Rosemary Conley Ready to Eat Porridge (available from chiller cabinet in Asda)

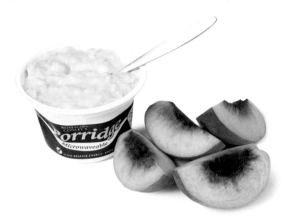

Mid-morning Power Snack

1 peach

Lunch

1 wholegrain or wholemeal tortilla wrap (max. 200 kcal) spread with 1 teaspoon sweet chilli sauce and filled with mixed salad leaves and 50g cooked chicken breast (no skin)

Mid-afternoon Power Snack

Vegetable crudités: ½ carrot, ¼ red pepper, ¼ green pepper, 1 stick celery, 1 × 5cm piece cucumber and 5 cherry tomatoes

Dinner

Haddock Lyonnaise (see recipe page 148) served with unlimited vegetables (excluding potatoes)

DAY 14

Breakfast
1 egg, boiled, served with 1 slice wholegrain bread, toasted, spread with Marmite, plus ½ fresh grapefruit

Mid-morning Power Snack
1 cereal bowl of mixed salad with oil-free dressing

Lunch ☑
Any prepacked sandwich of your choice (max. 5% fat and 250 kcal) plus 1 apple or orange

Mid-afternoon Power Snack
1 × 14g pack Asda organic mini raisins

Dinner
Pork and Chickpea Casserole (see recipe page 98) served with unlimited vegetables (excluding potatoes)

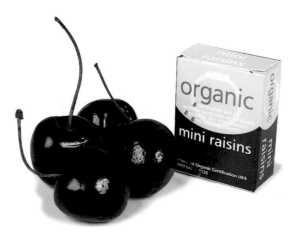

Slim to Win Diet: Week Three

Choose any breakfast, lunch or dinner from the following lists and, from week three, you can add on a treat, pudding and an alcoholic drink each day depending on your calorie allowance.

BREAKFASTS (approx. 200 calories each)

Fruit breakfasts
● Homemade fruit smoothie: blend 100g apricots, peaches or strawberries with 100g virtually fat-free fromage frais and 100ml milk from allowance
● Breakfast oat smoothie: in a blender, whizz 1 peach, 100g strawberries, 1 tablespoon oat bran and 100g low-fat plain or strawberry yogurt (max. 100 kcal and 5% fat) with enough milk from allowance to get desired consistency ☑
● ½ melon filled with 1 red portion pot/115g blueberries or raspberries, plus 1 low-fat fruit yogurt (max. 100 kcal and 5% fat) ☑
● Gi fruit salad: 1 satsuma, broken into segments, 1 chopped pear, 25g seedless grapes and 15g porridge oats mixed with 1 blue portion pot/80g 0% fat Greek yogurt
● 1 × 100g low-fat yogurt (max. 75 kcal and 5% fat) mixed with 1 sliced banana ☑
● 200g fresh fruit salad plus 100g low-fat yogurt (max. 5% fat) and 1 tablespoon muesli
● 1 × 175g pot Müller One a Day yogurt (any flavour) plus 1 yellow portion pot/70g blueberries

● 1 × 150g snack size pot Müller Rice, apple or strawberry flavour, plus 100g raspberries

Cereal breakfasts

● 1 Weetabix served with 100g canned peaches in natural juice, 100g low-fat natural yogurt and 1 teaspoon brown sugar ✓

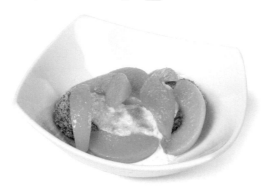

● Tropical muesli: 1 blue portion pot/40g muesli (max. 5% fat), topped with 30g each sliced kiwi fruit, mango, pineapple and melon and served with milk from allowance ✓
● 1 Weetabix or Shredded Wheat served with milk from allowance and 1 sliced banana ✓
● 1 blue portion pot/35g porridge oats made into porridge using water, served with milk from allowance and 1 teaspoon honey plus 1 peach ✓
● 1 green portion pot/50g Special K cereal served with milk from allowance and 5 sliced strawberries ✓
● 1 red portion pot/60g All-Bran served with milk from allowance and 1 teaspoon sugar ✓
● 1 red portion pot/50g branflakes or Sultana Bran served with milk from allowance and 1 teaspoon sugar ✓

● 2 Weetabix or Shredded Wheat served with milk from allowance and 1 teaspoon sugar ✓
● 1 red portion pot/30g Sugar Puffs served with milk from allowance and 1 low-fat fruit yogurt or fromage frais (max. 75 kcal and 5% fat) ✓
● 1 red portion pot/40g Special K served with milk from allowance and 150g mixed raspberries and blueberries ✓
● Blueberry crunch: 40g cornflakes, topped with 10g fresh blueberries, 2 tablespoons low-fat natural yogurt and 2 teaspoons maple syrup

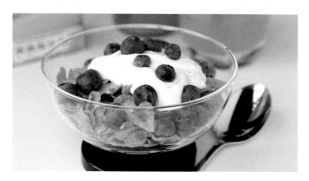

Cooked breakfasts

● 1 turkey rasher, grilled, 1 low-fat (max. 5% fat) sausage, grilled, plus 3 fresh tomatoes, grilled, and 1 yellow portion pot/115g baked beans
● 1 slice wholegrain bread, toasted, topped with 1 yellow portion pot/115g baked beans ✓
● 2 grilled turkey rashers served on 1 slice wholegrain bread, toasted, plus 1 small can (approx. 200g) tomatoes, boiled until reduced
● 1 poached or dry-fried egg served with 1 grilled low-fat sausage, 2 grilled tomatoes and 100g grilled mushrooms
● 1 boiled egg served with 1 slice wholegrain bread, toasted, spread with Marmite, plus ½ grapefruit ✓

● 50g smoked salmon served with 1 scrambled egg, plus ½ fresh grapefruit

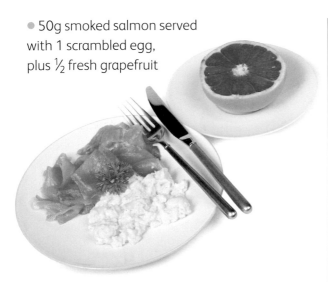

Quick breakfasts

● 1 slice wholegrain bread, toasted, spread with 1 teaspoon jam, marmalade or honey, plus 1 whole fresh grapefruit ☑

● Any Tasty Toast Topper (see recipes pages 168–169), plus 1 satsuma or clementine

● 1 crumpet, toasted, topped with 2 teaspoons jam or honey, 1 teaspoon 0% fat Greek-style yogurt and 5 raspberries ☑

● 1 mini bagel (60g), toasted, spread with 25g extra-light soft cheese and topped with 30g smoked salmon plus 1 apple

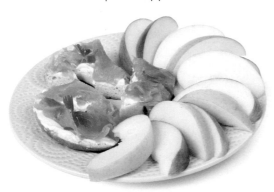

● 250ml any ready-made pure fruit smoothie (e.g. Innocent pure fruit strawberry and banana smoothie) plus 1 Alpen Light cereal bar any flavour (max. 200 kcal and 5% fat)

● 1 pot Rosemary Conley Ready to Eat Porridge (available from chiller cabinet in Asda) ☑

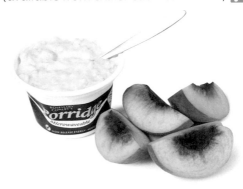

● 1 yellow portion pot/125ml fruit juice, plus 1 slice wholegrain bread, toasted, spread with 1 teaspoon jam, marmalade or honey ☑

● 1 Rosemary Conley Low Gi Nutrition Bar (from www.rosemaryconley.com) plus 1 yellow portion pot/125ml unsweetened fruit juice ☑

LUNCHES (approx. 300 calories each)

Sandwiches

● Any prepacked sandwich of your choice (max. 5% fat and 250 kcal) plus 1 apple or orange ☑

● 1 × 40g granary baguette spread with 20g extra-light soft cheese and topped with 25g wafer-thin ham or Quorn Deli Ham Style, plus 1 sliced tomato and chopped basil or chives ☑

● Spread 2 slices wholegrain bread with low-calorie salad dressing and make into an open sandwich with 40g low-fat cottage cheese or smoked salmon, topped with salad ☑

- 1 wholegrain or wholemeal tortilla wrap spread with 1 teaspoon cranberry sauce and 1 teaspoon extra-light mayonnaise, filled with 50g wafer-thin turkey or chicken and served with a small mixed salad
- 2 slices wholegrain bread spread with mustard or pickle, made into an open sandwich with 50g wafer-thin ham, chicken, turkey, plus a small salad served with oil-free dressing ☑
- 1 wholegrain or wholemeal tortilla wrap (max. 200 kcal) spread with 1 teaspoon sweet chilli sauce and filled with mixed salad leaves and 50g cooked chicken breast (no skin)
- 4 wholegrain Ryvitas topped with 60g (½ can) sardines in tomato sauce, mashed, plus a mixed salad tossed in oil-free dressing
- Lemon and Mustard Seed Houmous with Pitta (see recipe page 64) served with shredded lettuce leaves ☑

Salad lunches
- Any prepacked low-fat salad (max. 300 kcal and 5 % fat) ☑
- 1 × 250g pack ready-madeTuna Light Lunch tomato salsa flavour served with a small salad and 1 mini pitta bread
- Niçoise-style Beef Salad (see recipe page 81)
- Low-Gi rice salad: 1 blue portion pot/55g (uncooked weight) or 1 red portion pot/144g (cooked weight) boiled basmati rice, mixed with chopped spring onions, peppers, tomatoes, cucumber, mushrooms, tossed in soy sauce, served with 50g reduced-fat houmous or 25g wafer-thin chicken or turkey breast. Serve with mixed salad leaves

- Warm Chicken Caesar Salad (see recipe page 76)
- Balsamic Bean Salad (see recipe page 77) ☑
- 50g cooked or smoked salmon, mackerel or trout served with 1 teaspoon horseradish sauce and a large salad tossed in oil-free dressing
- 100g peeled, cooked prawns mixed with rocket leaves and sliced cucumber and drizzled with ½ teaspoon sweet chilli sauce served with 1 small (50g) wholemeal pitta bread
- 1 × 125g grilled chicken breast served with 1 blue portion pot/75g tomato salsa and a large mixed salad tossed in oil-free dressing, plus 1 kiwi fruit
- Large mixed salad (lettuce, tomato, peppers, celery, cucumber, carrot) and 75g drained canned tuna (in brine) mixed with 4 teaspoons extra-light mayonnaise and 2 chopped spring onions, plus 3 boiled new potatoes (with skins), cooled, then chopped and mixed with the tuna and salad
- Quick two bean salad: toss 100g each drained canned kidney beans and chickpeas, 1 sliced spring onion, 2 quartered cherry tomatoes, 1 celery stick, chopped red pepper and parsley in oil-free dressing; serve with 1 wholegrain crispbread spread with 1 tbsp half-fat cottage cheese ☑
- Fruity ham salad: 1 sliced peach, 100g cubed melon and 50g sliced ham served on a bed of mixed salad leaves tossed in oil-free dressing and served with 1 slice wholegrain bread
- Quick chicken Waldorf salad: 100g cooked chicken breast (no skin), diced, mixed with chopped celery, 1 chopped apple, chopped fresh

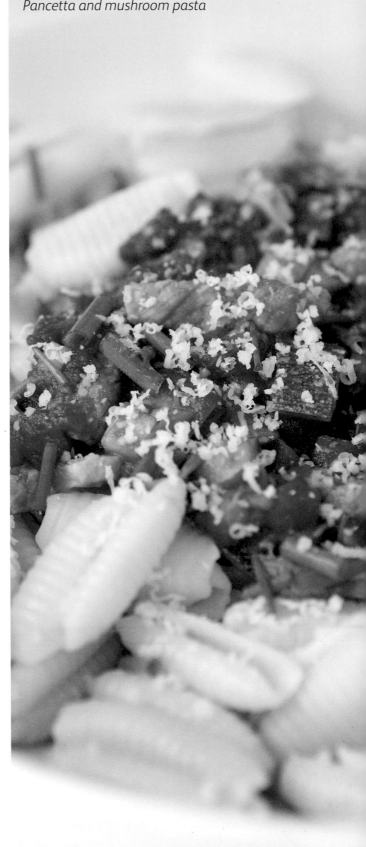

Pancetta and mushroom pasta

parsley and 4 tablespoons low-fat fromage frais and served with 2 rice cakes or 1 wholegrain Ryvita

Cooked lunches

- 2 slices wholegrain bread, toasted, topped with 1 yellow portion pot/115g baked beans ✔
- 1 small low-fat pizza (max. 230 kcal and 5 % fat) served with a large mixed salad tossed in oil-free dressing ✔
- 2 Quorn sausages, grilled, served with 1 yellow portion pot/100g mashed sweet potato plus boiled broccoli and cauliflower and low-fat gravy ✔
- 1 × 150g oven-baked sweet potato topped with any Jacket Potato Filler (see recipes pages 170–172), plus 1 piece fresh fruit (excluding bananas) ✔
- Piri Piri Chicken (see recipe page 74) served with a large mixed salad
- Pork and Pepper Fajitas (see recipe page 62)
- Any Tasty Toast Topper (see recipes pages 168–169) plus salad and 1 piece fresh fruit (excluding bananas) ✔
- Zesty Prawns (see recipe page 68) served with 115g boiled new potatoes (with skins) and unlimited green vegetables
- Three Pepper Pasta (see recipe page 123) ✔
- Pancetta and Mushroom Pasta (see recipe page 116)
- Sage Polenta with Chilli Tomatoes (see recipe page 70) served with salad ✔
- Mushroom and Saffron Pilaff (see recipe page 66) served with a large mixed salad, plus 1 low-fat yogurt (max. 100 kcal and 5 % fat) ✔

- Prawn Couscous (see recipe page 69) served with mixed salad leaves
- Quorn Stuffed Pepper (see recipe page 162) served with salad; 1 low-fat yogurt (max. 100 kcal and 5% fat) ☑

Soup lunches

- 1 × 400g can lentil or vegetable soup (max. 5% fat and 200 kcal) served with 1 slice toasted wholegrain bread ☑
- Leek and Sweet Potato Soup (see recipe page 52) served with 1 small wholegrain roll ☑
- Easy Pea and Ham Soup (see recipe page 54) served with 1 slice toasted wholegrain bread, plus 1 low-fat yogurt (max. 5% fat and 100 kcal)
- Vicky's Thai Coconut Noodle Soup (see recipe page 48) served with 1 slice wholegrain bread ☑

- Prawn Bisque (see recipe page 60) served with 1 small wholegrain roll
- Bortsch with Baby Vegetables (see recipe page 45) served with 1 small wholegrain roll ☑
- Tofu Rice Noodle Soup (see recipe page 58) ☑
- Thai Vegetable Soup (see recipe page 56) served with 1 small wholegrain roll, plus 1 apple or pear ☑
- Sun-Dried Tomato and Basil Soup (see recipe page 44), served with 1 small wholegrain roll, plus 1 apple or orange ☑

DINNERS (approx. 400 calories each)

Chicken and turkey dinners

- 1 × 115g chicken breast, grilled or baked, served with 1 × 150g oven-baked sweet potato and other vegetables of your choice
- 1 × 150g chicken breast (no skin) chopped and dry-fried until almost cooked. Add ½ pack stir-fry vegetables and unlimited beansprouts. When hot, add soy sauce and 1 tablespoon sweet chilli sauce
- Fruity Turkey Stir-Fry (see recipe page 88) served with 1 blue portion pot/55g (dry weight) or 1 red portion pot/144g (cooked weight) boiled basmati rice
- Chicken Enchiladas (see recipe page 194) served with red pepper salsa and green salad leaves
- Neil and Allyson's Speedy Chicken Curry (see recipe page 106) served with 40g (dry weight) boiled basmati rice
- Turkey Stir-Fry with Noodles (see recipe page 163)

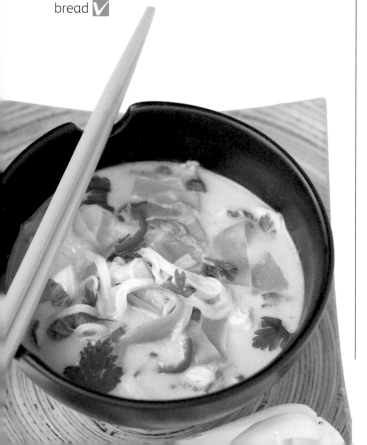

- Braised Turkey and Pork Rolls (see recipe page 133) served with 100g dry-roasted sweet potatoes, Courgette and Pepper Rosti (see recipe page 247) and green vegetables
- Tandoori Chicken Drumsticks (see recipe page 232) served with 1 blue portion pot/55g (dry weight) or 1 red portion pot/144g (cooked weight) boiled basmati rice and a green salad

Beef dinners
- Beef and Mushroom Crumble (see recipe page 138) served with unlimited vegetables (excluding tomatoes)
- Hearty Beef Casserole (see recipe page 102)
- Beef Pasanda (see recipe page 101) served with 1 blue portion pot/55g or 1 red portion pot/144g (cooked weight) boiled basmati rice
- Chilli Con Carne (see recipe page 139) served with 1 blue portion pot/55g (dry weight) or 1 red portion pot/144g (cooked weight) boiled basmati rice
- Beef and Broccoli Stir-Fry (see recipe page 91) served with 1 × 65g block (uncooked weight) boiled noodles
- Farfalle Bolognese (see recipe page 114) served with green salad
- Pan-Fried Beef with Brandy (see recipe page 174) served with 1 × 200g oven-baked sweet potato (with skin) or boiled new potatoes (with skins) and unlimited other vegetables

Pork dinners
- Pork and Pineapple Burgers (see recipe page 176) served in 1 wholegrain roll, plus tomato salsa and salad
- Pork Slices with Cheese and Sage (see recipe page 201) served with 1 blue portion pot/55g (dry weight) or 1 red portion pot/144g (cooked weight) boiled basmati rice, and salad
- Pork and Chickpea Casserole (see recipe page 98) served with unlimited vegetables (excluding potatoes)
- Pork with Balsamic Peppers and Noodles (see recipe page 175)
- Sweet and Sour Pork Chops (see recipe page 143) served with 75g boiled new potatoes (with skins) and unlimited green vegetables
- Chinese Pork Noodles (see recipe page 165)

Lamb dinners
- 115g lamb's liver braised in gravy and sliced onions, served with 115g boiled new potatoes (with skins) and unlimited other vegetables
- Lamb and Pepper Hotpot (see recipe page 134) served with green vegetables
- Lamb Cutlets with Garlic and Redcurrant Glaze (see recipe page 198) served with 75g boiled new potatoes (with skins) and green vegetables
- Pan-Fried Liver with Leek Mash (see recipe page 180) served with unlimited vegetables (excluding potatoes), plus 1 low-fat yogurt (max. 100 kcal and 5% fat)
- Teriyaki Lamb Skewers (see recipe page 199) served with 1 × 200g oven-baked sweet potato (with skin) and a mixed salad
- Navarin of Lamb (see recipe page 136) served with 175g boiled new potatoes (with skins) and unlimited other vegetables

Fish dinners

- 150g white fish, steamed, served with 115g boiled new potatoes (with skins) and steamed green vegetables
- 1 × 115g salmon steak, grilled, served with 115g boiled new potatoes (with skins) plus unlimited steamed green vegetables and 2 teaspoons low-calorie salad cream
- Baked Smoked Haddock with Peppers (see recipe page 204) served with 115g boiled new potatoes (with skins) and unlimited other vegetables or salad
- Fresh Tuna with Tomato and Radish Salsa (see recipe page 184) served with 1 blue portion pot/55g (uncooked weight) or 1 red portion pot/144g (cooked weight) boiled basmati rice
- Mussels with White Wine and Spinach (see recipe page 202) served with 1 slice wholegrain bread
- Haddock Lyonnaise (see recipe page 148) served with unlimited salad or vegetables (excluding potatoes)
- Seared Tuna with Balsamic Greens (see recipe page 186) served with 50g (uncooked weight) steamed couscous and a green salad tossed in oil-free dressing
- Fragrant Fish Curry (see recipe page 110) served with 1 blue portion pot/55g (uncooked weight) or 1 red portion pot/144g (cooked weight) boiled basmati rice

Vegetarian dinners

- 3 Quorn sausages, grilled, served with 115g mashed sweet potatoes, unlimited green vegetables and gravy ☑
- Garlic Baked Tomatoes (see recipe page 244) served with 1 × 200g oven-baked sweet potato and salad ☑
- Sweet Potato and Fennel Gratin (see recipe page 212) served with unlimited vegetables (excluding potatoes) or salad ☑
- Tomato and Cheese Tarts (see recipe page 235) served with 175g boiled new potatoes (with skins) and unlimited vegetables or salad ☑
- Mushroom and Spinach Pasta Bake (see recipe page 120) served with green salad ☑
- Quorn and Mushroom Stuffed Red Onions (see recipe page 151) served with 150g boiled new potatoes (with skins) and a salad ☑
- Falafels with Pitta and Yogurt (see recipe page 187) ☑
- Vegetable and Black Bean Noodle Stir-Fry (see recipe page 96) served with steamed pak choi or a mixed salad tossed in oil-free dressing, plus 1 low-fat yogurt (max. 75 kcal) ☑
- Quorn Lasagne Verde (see recipe page 128) plus a mixed leaf salad tossed in oil-free dressing; 1 satsuma ☑

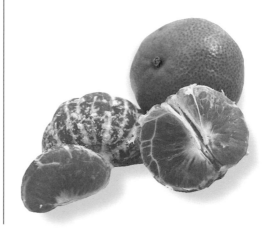

- Spinach and Ricotta Pie (see recipe page 208) served with tomato salad and 1 red portion pot/107g (cooked weight) or 1 blue portion pot/50g (dry weight) steamed couscous ☑
- Spicy Pasta with Rocket (see recipe page 167) ☑
- Veggie Cottage Pie (see recipe page 211) served with green vegetables or salad ☑
- Roweena's Healthy Pizza (see recipe page 124) served with salad or vegetables (excluding potatoes) ☑
- Basque Omelette (see recipe page 167) served with 150g boiled new potatoes (with skins) ☑

For more delicious meal ideas, see the recipe sections in this book and add accompaniments according to your personal calorie allowance (see pages 278–9).

POWER SNACKS

Choose two a day (approx. 50 calories each) and eat one mid-morning and mid-afternoon to stave off hunger pangs or combine two of them for an extra snack at any time of day.

- 12 seedless grapes
- 75g mango
- 200g melon (flesh only)
- 7 medium-sized strawberries
- 1 small or ½ large banana
- 1 apple or pear
- 2 satsumas
- 2 kiwi fruit
- 1 orange or nectarine
- 1 cereal bowl of mixed salad with oil-free dressing
- 3 ready to eat prunes
- 5 heaped tablespoons blueberries
- 3 dried apricots
- ½ medium grapefruit topped with 1 teaspoon raisins or sultanas
- 100g cherries
- 100g pomegranate seeds
- Tomato and basil salad: 2 tomatoes, sliced and mixed with 5 fresh basil leaves and ¼ red onion, finely chopped and lightly tossed in balsamic vinegar
- 5 mini low-fat breadsticks plus 1 tablespoon Total 0% fat Greek yogurt mixed with chopped chives
- Crudités with dip: 1 blue portion pot/75g tomato salsa, plus 5cm cucumber, 1 celery stick and ¼ yellow pepper, all cut into sticks
- 1 yellow portion pot/70g blueberries topped with 2 teaspoons Total 0% fat Greek yogurt
- 10 sweet silverskin pickled onions plus 10 cherry tomatoes
- Vegetable crudités: ½ carrot, ¼ red pepper, ¼ green pepper, 1 stick celery, 1 × 5cm piece cucumber and 5 cherry tomatoes
- 1 Kallo thick slice rice cake topped with 1 Laughing Cow Extra Light cheese triangle
- 1 × 90g Tesco Fresh Apple and Grape Snack Pack
- 1 Asda Good For You chicken noodle cup soup
- 1 Weight Watchers citrus fruit yogurt (pink grapefruit, lemon, or orange and nectarine)
- 1 × 14g pack Asda organic mini raisins

TREATS

From week three of the Slim to Win Diet you are allowed a daily treat. It can be anything you like, high fat or low fat, as long as it doesn't exceed 100 calories. All the ones listed below are under 100 calories and have 5% or less fat. If you want, you can save up your treats over seven days for a special occasion.

Lollies
- Wall's Mini Milk 31 kcal
- Del Monte Fruitini 44 kcal
- Wall's Mini Twister 46 kcal
- Rowntrees Fruit Pastil-lolly 60 kcal
- Wall's Mini Calippo 70 kcal
- The Skinny Cow Berry Blush smoothie 71 kcal
- Nestlé Fab lolly 79 kcal
- Del Monte Strawberry Fruit Double 83 kcal
- Del Monte Smoothie Mango 97 kcal
- The Skinny Cow Triple Chocolate 97 kcal

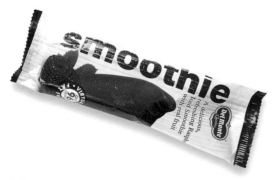

Cakes
- Morrisons Eat Smart lemon cake slice 81 kcal
- Mr Kipling Delightful apple slice 91 kcal
- Asda Good for You cherry bakewell slice 98 kcal
- Morrisons Eat Smart carrot cake slice 84 kcal
- Tesco Light Choices date and walnut cake slice 70 kcal
- Asda Good For You chocolate slice 95 kcal

Crisps
- 1 × 15g bag Asda Good For You sea salt and malt vinegar flavour potato fries 54 kcal
- 1 × 12g bag Morrisons Eat Smart diet bacon flavour waffle potato snack 42 kcal
- 1 × 20g bag Weight Watchers Mini Hoops salt and vinegar flavour 70 kcal
- 1 × 10g bag Morrisons Eat Smart diet pickled onion ring flavour potato snack 35 kcal
- 25g Penn State Pretzels original salted 94 kcal

Cereal and snack bars
- Asda Good For You pomegranate cereal bar 76 kcal
- Alpen Light chocolate and orange bars 60 kcal
- Alpen light summer fruits 59 kcal
- Ryvita Goodness Bar apple and sultana flavour 62 kcal
- Jordans Frusli All Fruit strawberry bar 94 kcal

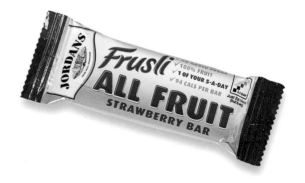

ALCOHOLIC DRINKS

All these alcoholic drinks are under 100 calories. Use slimline mixers and diet drinks with spirits to keep the calories down.

Beer
- 300ml/½ pint bitter 91 kcal
- 300ml/½ pint lager 82 kcal

Brandy and liqueurs
- 1 × 25ml measure brandy 50 kcal
- 1 × 25ml measure Southern Comfort 81 kcal
- 1 × 25ml measure Tia Maria 75 kcal

Sprits
- 1 × 25ml measure Bacardi 56 kcal
- 1 × 275ml bottle Diet Bacardi Breezer 96 kcal
- 1 × 25ml measure gin 50 kcal
- 1 × 25ml measure vodka 50 kcal
- 1 × 25ml measure whisky 50 kcal

Vermouth
- 1 × 50ml measure Martini Rosso 70 kcal
- 1 × 50ml measure Martini Extra Dry 48 kcal

Wine and fortified wine
- 1 × 125ml glass champagne 95 kcal
- 1 × 125ml glass dry white wine 83 kcal
- 1 × 125ml glass medium white wine 93 kcal
- 1 × 125ml glass red wine 85 kcal
- 1 × 125ml glass medium rosé wine 89 kcal
- 1 × 50ml measure port 79 kcal
- 1 × 50ml measure sweet sherry 68 kcal
- 1 × 50ml measure dry sherry 58 kcal

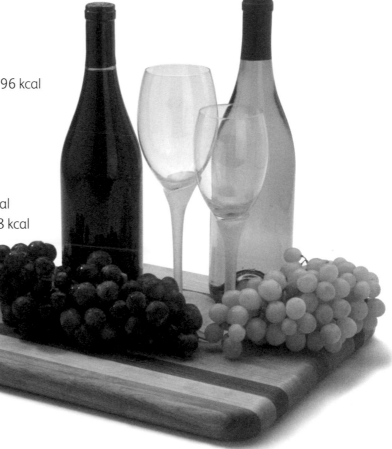

Clever cooking

To cook the low-fat way you'll need to invest in some non-stick pans and baking tins and learn how to minimise the fat content of recipes without compromising the taste.

How to dry-fry foods

Dry-frying is a key low-fat cooking method that does away with the need to use oil. The trick is to have your non-stick pan over the correct heat. If it's too hot, the pan will dry out too soon and the contents will burn; if the heat is too low, you lose the crispness recommended for a stir-fry. A simple rule is to preheat the empty pan until it is hot (but not too hot) before adding the ingredients. Test if the pan is hot enough by adding a piece of meat or fish (or whatever you'll be cooking). If it sizzles on contact, then the pan is at the right temperature. Once the meat is sealed on all sides (when it changes colour) you can reduce the heat a little as you add other ingredients.

Cooking meat and poultry is simple, as the natural fat and juices run out almost immediately, providing plenty of moisture to prevent burning. When cooking minced meat it's best to dry-fry it first and then place in a colander to drain any fat that has emerged. Wipe out the pan with a wad of kitchen paper to remove any fatty residue before continuing to cook your shepherd's pie or bolognese sauce.

Vegetables contain their own juices and soon release them when they become hot, so dry-frying vegetables works well, too. It is important not to overcook them, though. They should be crisp and colourful so that they retain their flavour and most of their nutrients.

Occasionally you may wish to add a little low-calorie cooking spray oil to line your pan or baking tin as this aids the cooking or baking of dishes such as 'fried' eggs, fish, cakes, Yorkshire puddings, and so on. Use sparingly.

Flavour enhancers

It's important to add moisture and extra flavour to compensate for the lack of oil or fat. Wine, soy sauce, wine vinegar, and even fresh lemon juice all provide liquid in which food can be 'fried' or cooked. However, some thicker types of sauces can dry out too fast if they are added early on in cooking, so add them later when there is more moisture in the pan.

Adding freshly ground black pepper to just about any savoury dish is a real flavour enhancer. You will need a good pepper mill and, ideally, you should buy peppercorns whole and in large quantities. Ready-ground black pepper is nowhere near as good.

When cooking rice, pasta and vegetables, add a vegetable stock cube to the cooking water. Although stock cubes do contain some fat, the amount absorbed by the food is negligible and the benefit in flavour is noticeable. Always save the cooking water from vegetables to make soups, gravy and sauces.

Make swaps
Here is a quick reference list of ingredients that can be substituted for traditional high-fat ones:

Cheese sauce Make by using a small amount of low-fat cheddar or Rosemary Conley's Mature Cheese (available in Asda and Morrisons), a little made-up mustard and skimmed milk mixed with a little cornflour.

Custard Use custard powder and follow the instructions on the packet, substituting skimmed milk and artificial sweetener for sugar to save calories.

Cream Instead of double cream or whipping cream, use 0% fat Greek yogurt or fromage frais towards the end of cooking but do not boil. Instead of single cream, use natural or vanilla-flavoured yogurt or fromage frais.

Cream cheese Use Quark (low-fat skimmed soft cheese) or Philadelphia Extra Light soft cheese.

Roux To make a low-fat roux, add dry, plain flour to the pan containing the other ingredients to thicken the sauce and then 'cook out' the flour, then slowly add liquid. Alternatively, use cornflour mixed with cold water or milk, bring to the boil and cook for 2–3 minutes.

Thickening for sweet sauces Arrowroot, slaked in cold water or juice, is a good thickener because it becomes translucent when cooked.

Herbs

Herbs can be added to virtually any dish. Dried herbs are more strongly flavoured than fresh, although it's usually better to use fresh herbs where possible as some nutrients are lost during the drying process. As a general rule, 1 teaspoon of dried herbs equals 4 teaspoons of fresh. Herbs are usually added in the last few minutes of cooking. Parsley, however, retains its flavour during cooking and can be added at the start.

Here are some guidelines on using herbs:

Basil Add to tomato soup, potato dishes, meat, poultry, pasta, rice and egg dishes.

Bay Use in soups, stews, casseroles, meat and poultry marinades and stocks.

Chives Sprinkle on salads and dressings, chicken, soups and egg dishes.

Dill Good with salads, fish, cheese and potato dishes.

Lemongrass Goes well with stir-fries, curries, seafood and soups.

Marjoram Add to meat, fish and egg and cheese dishes.

Mint Add to meat, chicken, sauces and vegetable dishes.

Oregano Good in stuffings and pasta, egg and cheese dishes.

Parsley Use in salads, sauces, seafood, pasta, rice and egg and vegetable dishes.

Rosemary Goes well with fish, poultry, meat, sauces and soups.

Sage Add to stuffings and tomato and cheese dishes.

Tarragon Use in salad dressings and egg dishes.

Thyme Good in stuffings, poultry dishes, soups, stocks and stews.

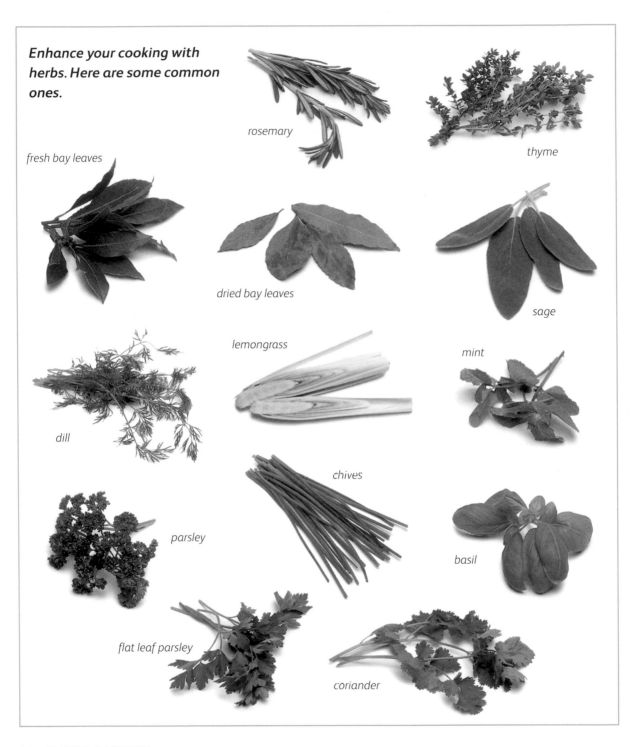

Enhance your cooking with herbs. Here are some common ones.

rosemary

thyme

fresh bay leaves

dried bay leaves

sage

lemongrass

mint

dill

chives

parsley

basil

flat leaf parsley

coriander

Spices

There are many varieties of blended spice mixes to add heat and flavour to meat and vegetable dishes. These are great for a quick and easy curry sauce, although many of the individual spice flavours are lost during the blending. Using one or two spices to flavour food rather than a blend adds a more distinctive delicate flavour.

As spices need to be cooked out in order to obtain the maximum favour, always start by dry-frying spices in a wok or infusing the spice in the cooking liquor for 2–3 minutes before adding the main ingredient.

Here are some great spice combinations:

Cardamom whole pods Use 4–5 to rice or vegetables during cooking.

Cumin seeds lightly toasted Add a pinch to cooked carrots or root vegetables.

Coriander seeds lightly toasted Use in salads whole or crush for sauces.

Mustard seed lightly toasted Goes well with potatoes or use as a seasoning for fish.

Saffron Soak in 2 tablespoons of boiling water for 5 minutes. Add to cooked rice or stir into yogurt.

Nutmeg Coarsely grate directly into a hot wok containing vegetables.

Fennel or Fenugreek seeds lightly toasted Add to cauliflower during cooking.

Marinades

A low-fat marinade can enhance the flavour of meat, fish and poultry. You can use it to baste meat or fish during cooking or pour it over in advance and leave for a couple of hours or overnight. The latter method is ideal for casseroles.

If you use salt, add it during cooking, not before, as it will draw out the juices from the meat if added at the marinade stage. Try these simple marinades:

Pork Pineapple juice thickened with tomato purée and a little ground cinnamon.

Beef Rich soy sauce mixed with a little horseradish sauce and crushed green peppercorns.

Lamb Heated redcurrant jelly or cranberry sauce mixed with a little soy sauce. When cooked, sprinkle with chopped fresh mint.

Poultry Chopped fresh ginger mixed with fresh orange juice and then thickened with a little runny honey.

Fish Toss the fish in a combination of fresh herbs such as chives, parsley and coriander. Drizzle with lemon juice and light soy sauce before cooking.

Vegetarian Finely diced red onion mixed with 2 tablespoons of light soy sauce, 1 crushed garlic clove and 2 tablespoons of apple sauce.

Ten quick tips for low-fat cooking

1 Always use cooking pans or woks with non-stick surfaces.

2 When stirring or preparing food in a non-stick pan use wooden spoons, spatulas or other non-stick utensils.

3 Always preheat your pan to 'hot' before adding your meat, poultry, fish or vegetables. Test the temperature by adding a piece. If it sizzles, the pan is hot enough.

4 Use wine, soy sauce and balsamic vinegar in stir-fries and salads in place of oil.

5 Remove all visible fat and skin from chops, joints, chicken, etc. before cooking.

6 To dry-roast potatoes and parsnips, peel then cut in half or quarters. Cook in boiling water with a vegetable stock cube for 5 minutes. Drain, then place on a non-stick baking tray and cook in the top of the oven – 45 minutes for potatoes, 30 minutes for parsnips – until golden brown.

7 Make gravy with vegetable water and low-fat granules or gravy powder.

8 Add a vegetable stock cube when cooking rice, pasta or vegetables. It gives a delicious flavour and removes the need to add butter or oil before serving.

9 Use 0% fat Greek-style yogurt or virtually fat-free fromage frais instead of cream to flavour dishes.

10 When using yogurt or fromage frais in cooking never allow them to boil, or they will curdle.

Note: while salt is often included in the recipes in this book, you may choose to omit it for health reasons.

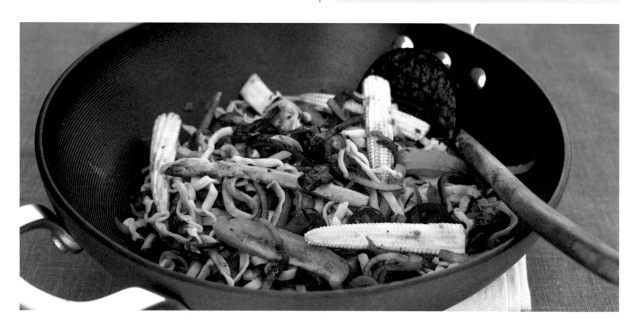

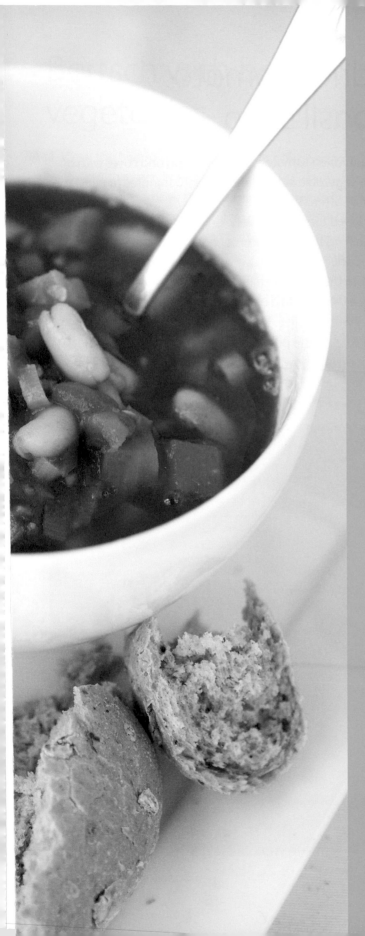

Soups

There's nothing more comforting than a bowl of soup, and homemade ones taste best. Add a chunk of crusty wholegrain bread for a simple but satisfying lunch, or serve up as a dinner party starter.

Vicky's Thai coconut noodle soup

SERVES 4
PER SERVING
196 CALORIES
4.1G FAT

PREPARATION TIME 5 MINUTES
COOKING TIME 10 MINUTES

600ml vegetable stock
200g Thai rice noodles
½ red onion, finely chopped
2 smoked garlic cloves, crushed
1 teaspoon lemongrass paste
1 teaspoon finely chopped fresh
    ginger
1 small red chilli, sliced
1 large carrot, sliced
2 celery sticks, finely sliced
100g mushrooms, sliced
100ml reduced-fat coconut milk
100g pak choi, sliced
fresh parsley to garnish

TIP *Freeze any leftover
coconut milk*

1 Bring the vegetable stock to the boil in a large saucepan. When boiling, add the noodles and cook for 5 minutes.
2 Meanwhile, heat a non-stick wok, and dry-fry the onion and garlic until soft. Add the lemongrass paste, ginger, chilli, carrot, celery and mushrooms, tossing them well together.
3 Pour the coconut milk into the wok, then add the noodles and their stock. Cook until the noodles are soft, then add the pak choi and ladle into serving bowls. Garnish with fresh parsley.

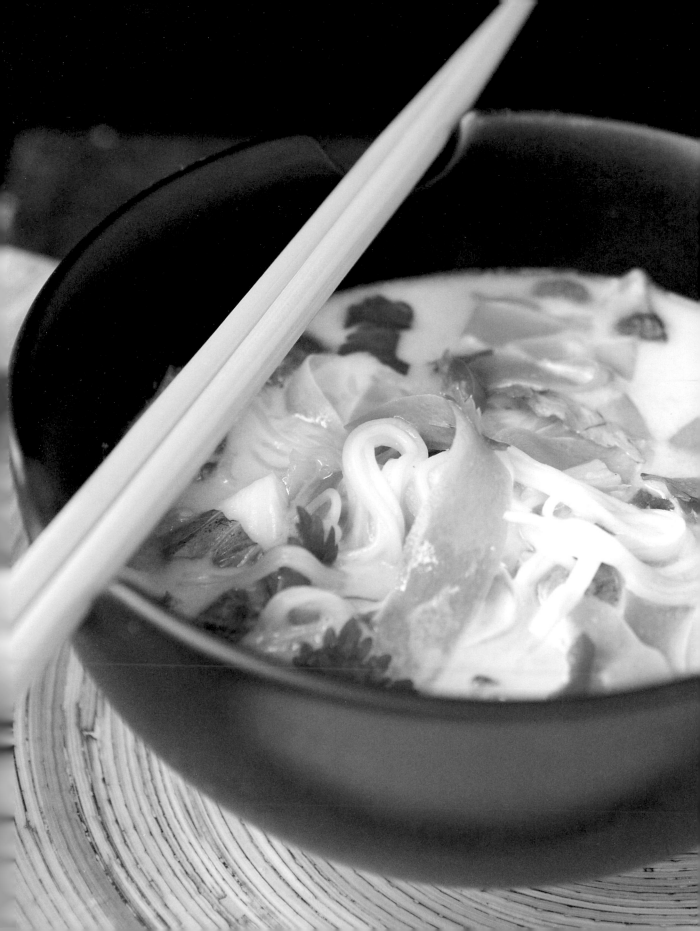

Double pepper soup with chive cream

SERVES 4
PER SERVING
141 CALORIES
1.8G FAT

PREPARATION TIME 20 MINUTES
COOKING TIME 30 MINUTES

4 red peppers, deseeded and
   chopped
4 yellow peppers, deseeded
   and chopped
2 celery sticks, sliced
2 medium onions, chopped
2 garlic cloves, crushed
2 teaspoons chopped fresh
   lemon or common thyme
2 litres vegetable stock
2 bay leaves
salt and freshly ground black
   pepper

for the chive cream
2 tablespoons virtually fat free
   fromage frais
1 tablespoon finely chopped
   chives
salt and freshly ground black
   pepper

TIP *The soup, but not the chive cream, is ideal for freezing*

1. Put the red and the yellow peppers in 2 separate saucepans. Divide the celery, onions, garlic and thyme between each pan, then add half the vegetable stock and bay leaves to each pan. Bring to the boil and simmer gently until the vegetables are soft.
2. Remove the bay leaves and liquidise each soup separately until smooth, rinsing out the liquidiser between soups. Adjust the consistency with a little extra stock if required and season with salt and freshly ground black pepper.
3. Return each soup to its original pan to reheat.
4. For the chive cream, mix together the fromage frais and chives and season with salt and freshly ground black pepper.
5. To serve, pour equal quantities of each soup into 2 identical jugs. Holding a jug in each hand at either side of a soup bowl, pour both soups into the bowl. Garnish with the chive cream.

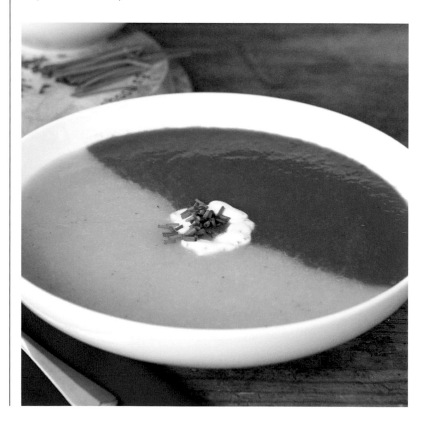

Cream of chicken soup

1 Heat a large non-stick saucepan. Add the chicken, celery, onion and garlic and dry-fry for 2–3 minutes.
2 Pour in a little stock, then sprinkle over the flour and mix well. Cook out the flour for 1 minute before gradually mixing in the remaining stock and then the milk.
3 Simmer gently for 10–15 minutes to allow the soup to thicken. Stir in the parsley. Just before serving, remove from the heat and stir in the yogurt. Garnish with a few chives.

SERVES 4 PER SERVING
137 CALORIES
3.3G FAT

PREPARATION TIME 10 MINUTES
COOKING TIME 20 MINUTES

1 × 175g skinless chicken
    breast, cut into small pieces
2 celery sticks, finely chopped
1 onion, finely chopped
2 garlic cloves, crushed
300ml vegetable stock
1 tablespoon plain flour
300ml semi-skimmed milk
1 tablespoon chopped fresh
    parsley
2 tablespoons low-fat yogurt
chopped chives to garnish

TIP *Try adding some canned or frozen sweetcorn to this rich soup*

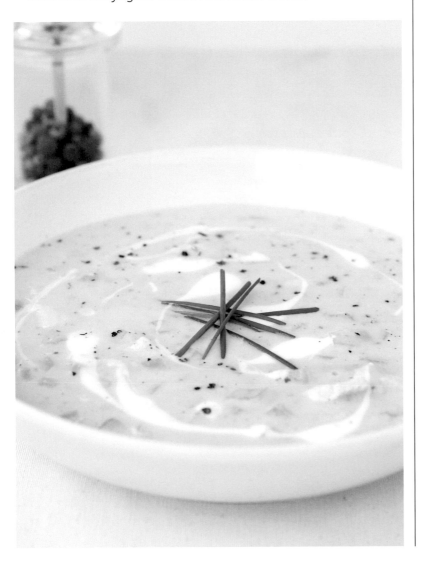

Leek and sweet potato soup

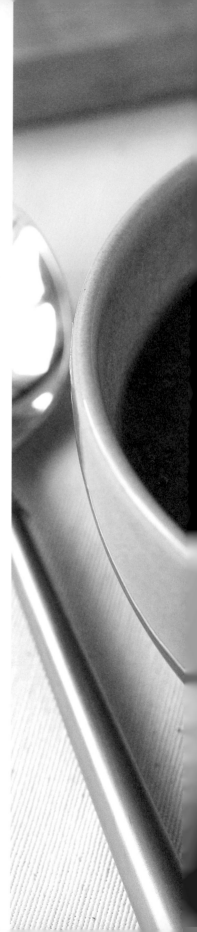

SERVES 4
PER SERVING
136 CALORIES
1.3G FAT

PREPARATION TIME 10 MINUTES
COOKING TIME 30 MINUTES

2 medium-sized leeks, chopped
2 garlic cloves, crushed
1 tablespoon chopped fresh
   thyme
2 sweet potatoes, peeled and
   chopped
1.2 litres vegetable stock
2 bay leaves
1 tablespoon tomato purée
salt and freshly ground black
   pepper
fresh parsley to garnish

TIP *You can add a blob of
virtually fat-free fromage frais
on top or sprinkle with a little
grated fresh nutmeg*

1 Heat a heavy-based, non-stick pan, and dry-fry the leeks until soft. Add the garlic and continue cooking for 1–2 minutes. Add the thyme and sweet potatoes, then pour in the stock.

2 Add the bay leaves and tomato purée, and simmer gently until the potatoes are cooked.

3 Remove the bay leaves and discard. Pour the soup into a liquidiser or blender and liquidise until smooth.

4 Return the soup to the pan and reheat. Adjust the consistency with a little extra stock. Season to taste and serve hot or cold garnished with fresh parsley.

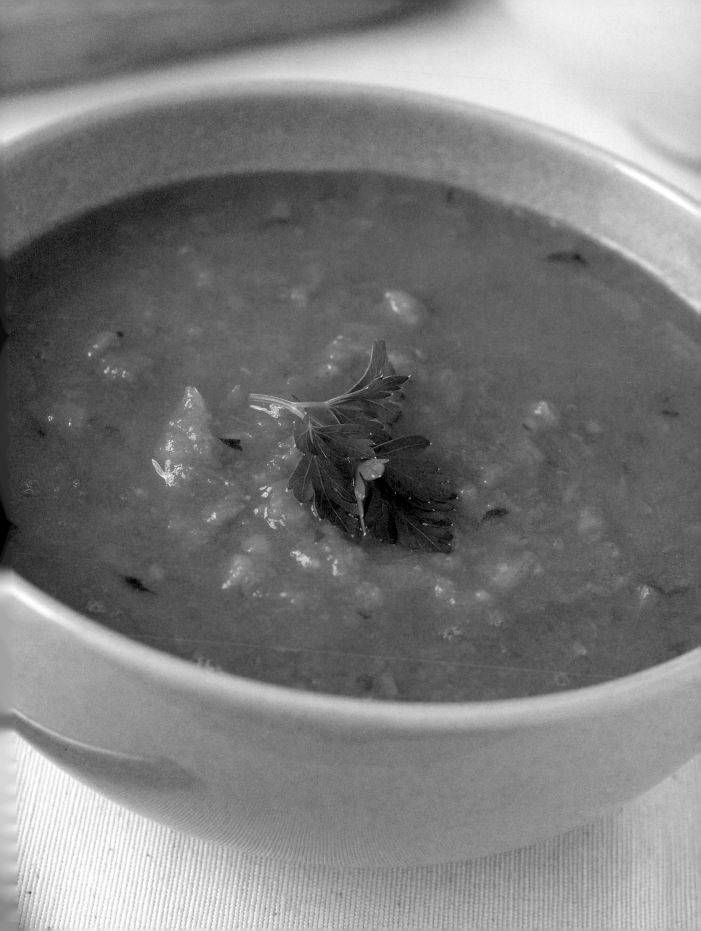

Easy pea and ham soup

❄

SERVES 4
PER SERVING
102 CALORIES
1.9G FAT

PREPARATION TIME 10 MINUTES
COOKING TIME 15 MINUTES

450g frozen peas
8 spring onions, chopped
2 garlic cloves, crushed
600ml vegetable stock
juice of ½ lemon
2 slices (50g) lean cooked ham
chopped fresh parsley
2 tablespoons low-fat natural
    yogurt

TIP *For a minty-flavoured
soup use frozen minted peas*

1 Put the frozen peas, spring onions, garlic and vegetable stock
   into a large saucepan. Bring to the boil and simmer for 10
   minutes.
2 Pour the soup into a food processor, add the lemon juice and
   blend until smooth.
3 Return the soup to the pan and adjust the consistency, adding a
   little more stock if required.
4 Cut the ham into thin strips, add to the soup and heat through.
   Just before serving stir in some chopped fresh parsley and swirl
   the yogurt on top.

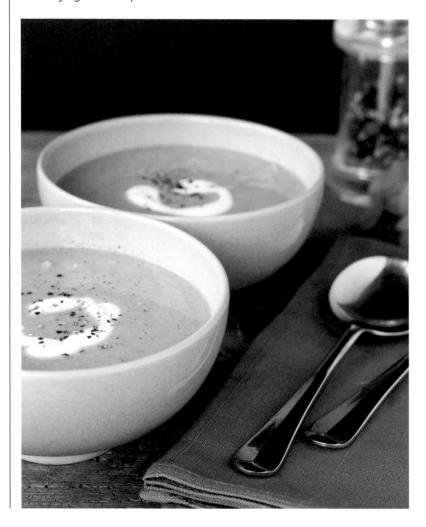

Three bean soup

1 Rinse the beans and put in a large saucepan. Add the vegetable stock and bring to the boil.
2 Heat a non-stick frying pan, and dry-fry the bacon (if using), shallots, garlic and celery for 5–6 minutes until soft. Transfer to the saucepan and add the thyme. Reduce the heat and simmer gently for 10 minutes.
3 Ladle half the soup into a food processor and blend until smooth. Return to the saucepan and adjust the consistency of the soup to your requirements with a little skimmed milk.
4 Season well with black pepper and serve hot.

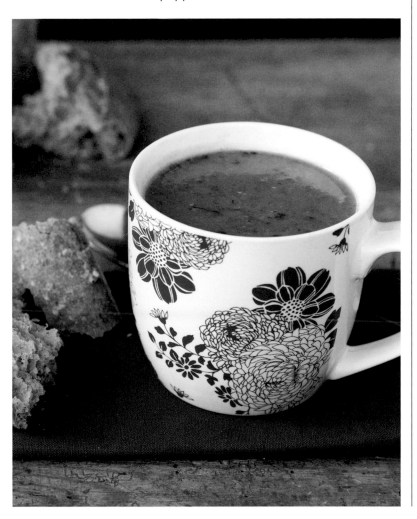

SERVES 6
PER SERVING
251 CALORIES
2.1G FAT

PREPARATION TIME 15 MINUTES
COOKING TIME 30 MINUTES

1 × 400g can kidney beans
1 × 400g can cannellini beans
1 × 400g can pinto beans, rinsed
1 litre vegetable stock
4 rashers smoked lean back bacon, cut into strips (optional)
4 small shallots, finely chopped
2 garlic cloves, crushed
2 celery sticks, chopped
2 teaspoons chopped fresh thyme
150ml skimmed milk
freshly ground black pepper

TIP *Processing just half the soup thickens it without making it completely smooth*

Thai vegetable soup

SERVES 4
PER SERVING
71 CALORIES
1.5G FAT

PREPARATION TIME 15 MINUTES
SOAKING TIME (BEANS) OVERNIGHT
COOKING TIME 1 HOUR

50g white beans (cannellini or
   haricot), soaked overnight
4 small shallots, finely chopped
2 garlic cloves, crushed
4 large carrots, diced
3 celery sticks, finely sliced
1 × 4cm piece lemongrass,
   finely sliced
1 × 2cm piece fresh ginger,
   finely chopped
2 × 400g cans chopped
   tomatoes
2–3 teaspoons vegetable stock
   bouillon powder, or to taste
freshly ground black pepper

TIP *Make this soup a day in
advance to allow the flavours
to develop*

1 After soaking the beans overnight,
   rinse well and place in a large
   saucepan with the shallots, garlic,
   carrots and celery. Cover with water
   and bring to the boil. Reduce the
   heat and simmer gently for 30
   minutes, topping up with water as
   required.
2 Add the lemongrass, ginger and
   tomatoes. Taste the soup and stir
   in the stock powder, adjusting the
   consistency with more water if
   necessary. Simmer for a further 25
   minutes until the beans are soft.
3 Season with black pepper and
   serve hot.

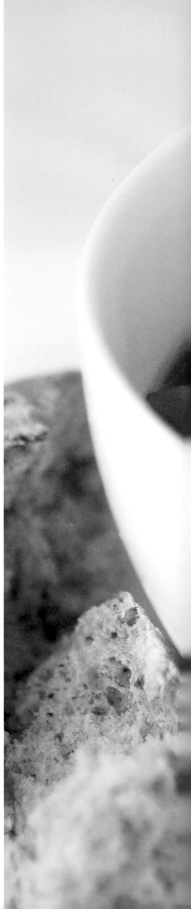

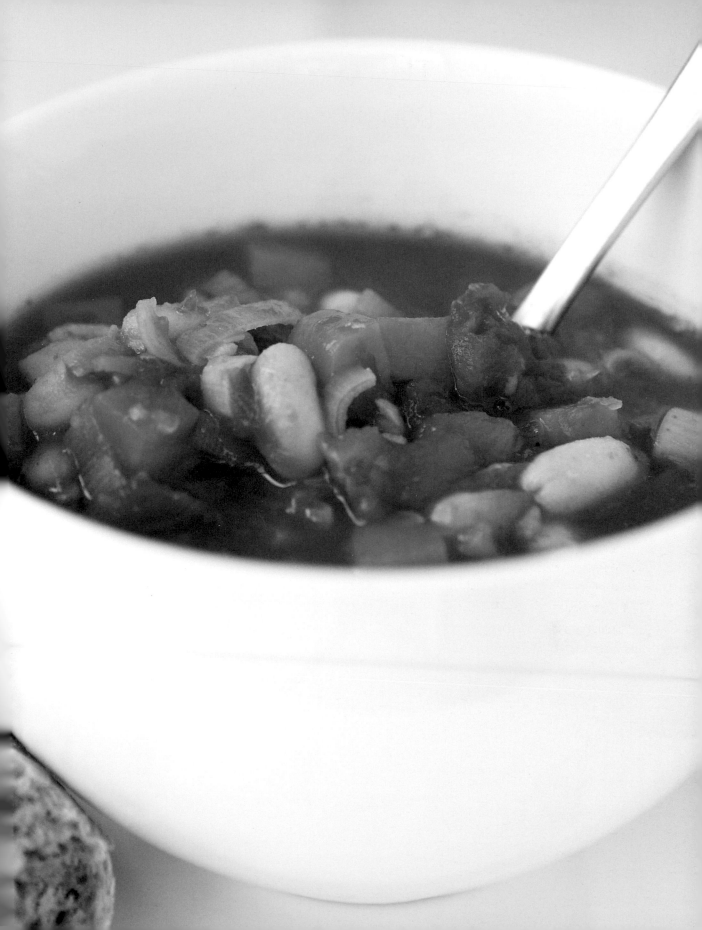

Tofu rice noodle soup

SERVES 4
PER SERVING
292 CALORIES
9G FAT

PREPARATION TIME 25 MINUTES
COOKING TIME 30 MINUTES

200g tofu
6 spring onions, finely chopped
1 garlic clove, crushed
2 teaspoons ground coriander
½ teaspoon ground turmeric
¼ teaspoon fenugreek seeds or
   ground fenugreek
1 small fresh red chilli, chopped
seeds from 4 crushed
   cardamom pods
4 Kaffir lime leaves (optional)
600ml vegetable stock
100g fine rice noodles
2 tablespoons chopped fresh
   basil
50g shredded fresh spinach
freshly ground black pepper

1 Preheat a non-stick wok or frying pan. Cut the tofu into cubes and drain on kitchen paper. Dry-fry the tofu until lightly browned on all sides, and season with black pepper.
2 Place all the remaining ingredients except the basil and spinach in a large saucepan and bring to a gentle simmer.
3 When the noodles are cooked, add the tofu, basil and spinach and heat through.
4 Remove the soup from the heat and serve hot.

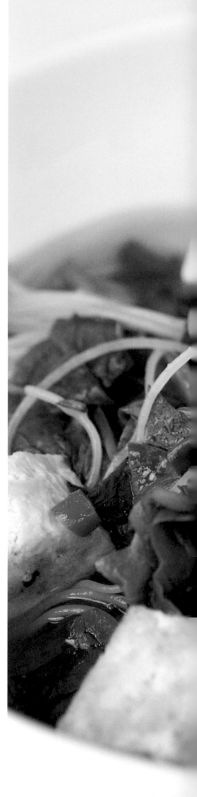

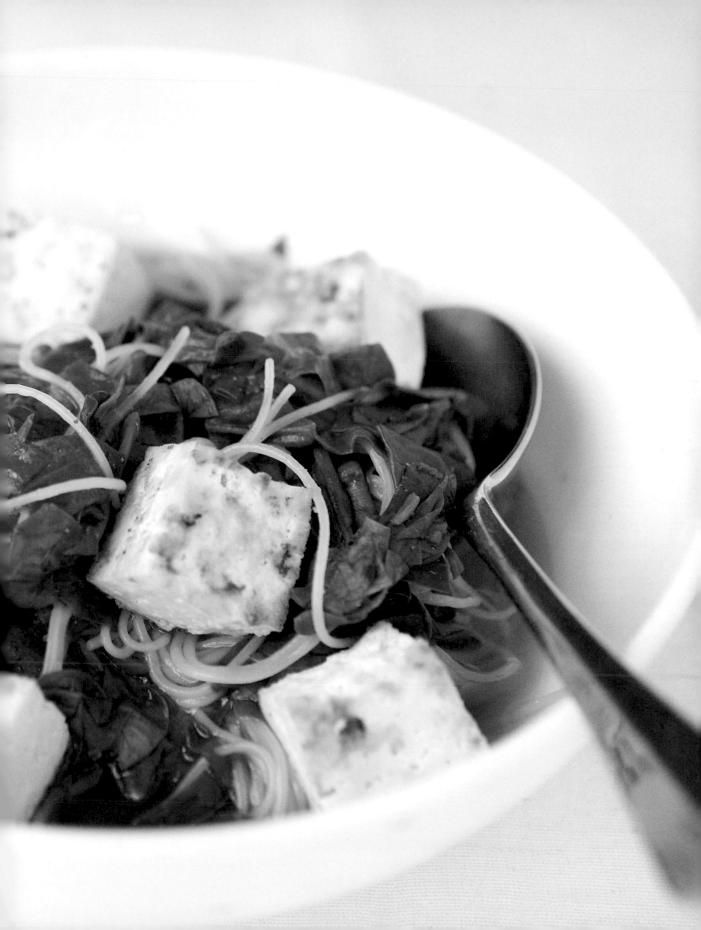

Prawn bisque

SERVES 4
PER SERVING
151 CALORIES
1.4G FAT

PREPARATION TIME 10 MINUTES
COOKING TIME 25 MINUTES

2 red large onions, chopped
2 garlic cloves, crushed
2 celery sticks, chopped
600ml fish or vegetable stock
150ml dry sherry
225g cooked prawns
1 teaspoon anchovy paste
2 tablespoons tomato purée
salt and freshly ground black
    pepper
2 tablespoons low-fat natural
    yogurt to serve

for the garnish
4 large cooked prawns
fresh dill

TIP *As the prawns need to be eaten fresh this soup is not suitable for freezing*

1   Heat a large, non-stick saucepan, add the onions, garlic and celery and dry-fry until soft.
2   Add the remaining ingredients except the yogurt and simmer gently for 5 minutes. Pour into a food processor and blend until smooth. Return to the pan and adjust the seasoning.
3   Just before serving stir in the low-fat yogurt. Spoon into serving bowls and garnish each with a large prawn and some fresh dill.

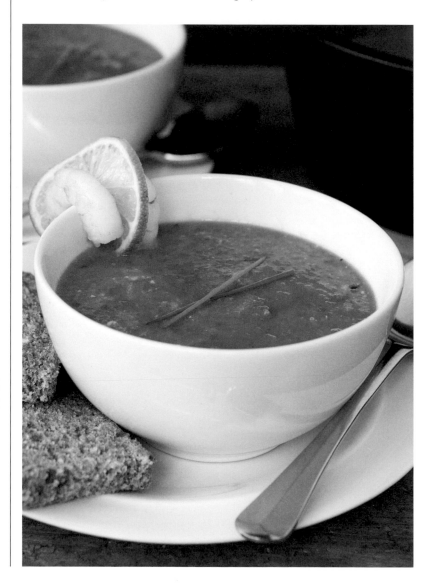

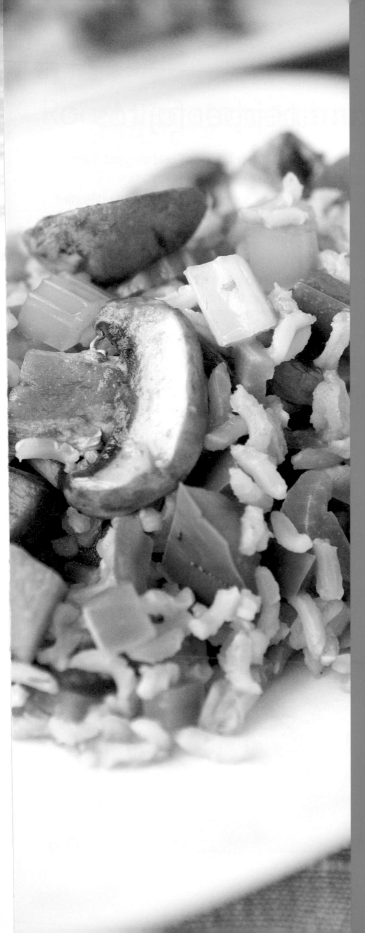

Light lunches

If you are having your main meal in the evening these recipes will help fill you up in the middle of the day without filling you out! If served cold, they also make ideal picnic or lunchbox food.

Lemon and mustard seed houmous with pitta

SERVES 4
PER SERVING
148 CALORIES
4.7G FAT

PREPARATION TIME 10 MINUTES
COOKING TIME 15 MINUTES

1 × 425g can chickpeas with no
    added salt or sugar
300ml soya milk
2 garlic cloves, crushed
2 teaspoons mustard seed
juice of ½ lemon
salt and cayenne pepper to
    taste
4 mini pitta breads to serve

1 Drain and rinse the chickpeas and place in a food processor.
2 Add the milk, garlic and mustard seed and process until smooth.
   Season with salt and pepper, add the lemon juice, then blend
   again to combine. Gradually pour in the milk, adjusting the
   consistency to a smooth paste and adjust the seasoning to
   taste.
3 Toast the pitta breads or warm in a microwave and serve with
   the houmous dip.

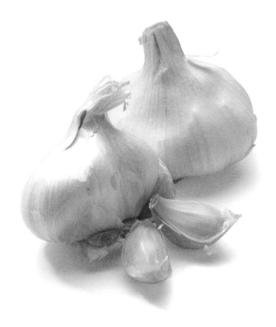

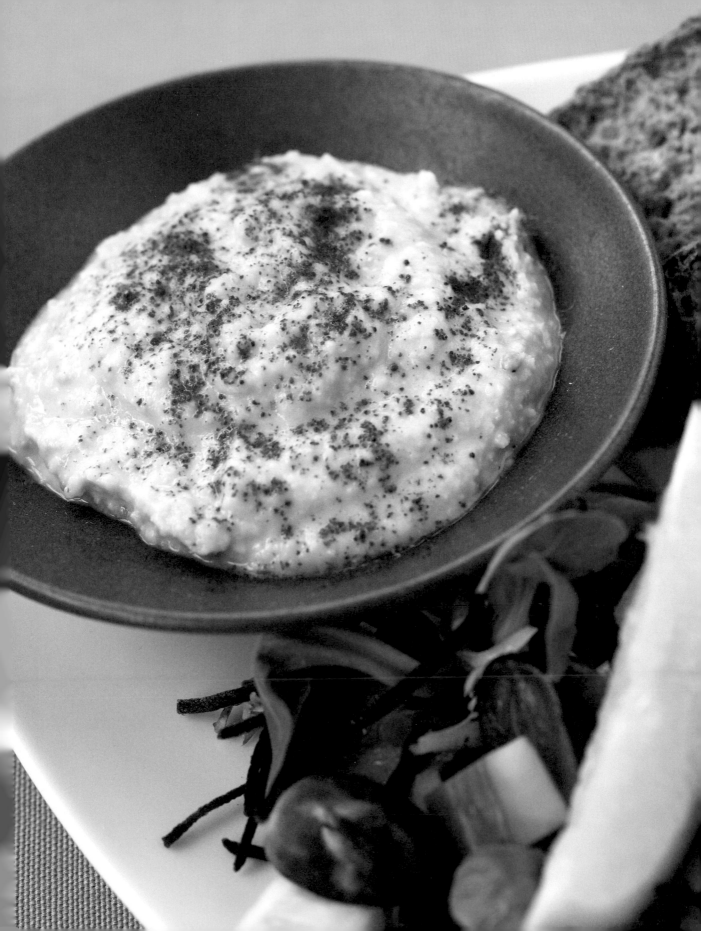

Mushroom and saffron pilaff

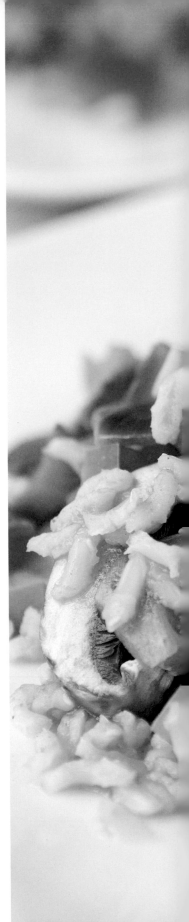

PER SERVING
SERVES 4
141 CALORIES
1G FAT

PREPARATION TIME 20 MINUTES
COOKING TIME 30 MINUTES

1 small red onion, finely
   chopped
1 celery stick, finely sliced
1 small green pepper, deseeded
   and finely diced
225g chestnut mushrooms,
   sliced
1 garlic clove, crushed
100g (dry weight) brown
   basmati rice
600ml vegetable stock
pinch of saffron strands
1 teaspoon chopped fresh
   thyme
100g frozen peas
freshly ground black pepper

TIP *Wash the rice well under
running water before adding
to the wok. This removes the
starch so that the rice doesn't
stick together once cooked*

1 Heat a non-stick wok, and dry-fry the
  onion, celery, green pepper,
  mushrooms and garlic over a high
  heat for 4–5 minutes, stirring
  occasionally.
2 Add the rice, stock, saffron and
  thyme. Stir well, then simmer gently
  to allow the liquid to be absorbed.
3 When ready to serve, season with
  black pepper to taste and stir in the
  frozen peas. Allow them to heat
  through before serving. Serve with a
  large mixed salad.

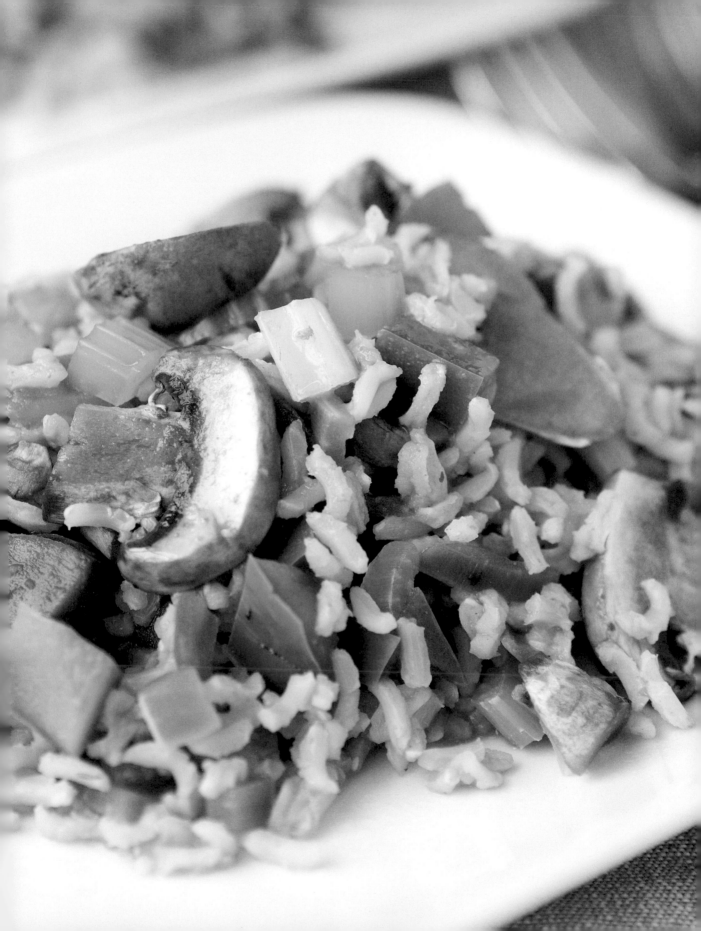

Zesty prawns

1 Heat a non-stick wok or frying pan, and dry-fry the onion and garlic for 3–4 minutes or until soft without colour.
2 Add the mushrooms and prawns and, as the prawns start to colour, pour in the tomato passata, then add the lemon zest and juice and chopped chives.
3 Bring the sauce to the boil, then check if the prawns are cooked, and season with salt and black pepper.
4 Serve with boiled rice and steamed green vegetables.

※

PER SERVING
SERVES 4
136 CALORIES
1.4G FAT

PREPARATION TIME 10 MINUTES
COOKING TIME 10 MINUTES

1 small white onion, finely chopped,
1 garlic clove, crushed
225g chestnut mushrooms
175g uncooked prawns
1 × 500g packet tomato passata
zest and juice of 1 lemon
1 tablespoon chopped fresh chives
salt and freshly ground black pepper

TIP *Don't overcook the prawns or they will become tough*

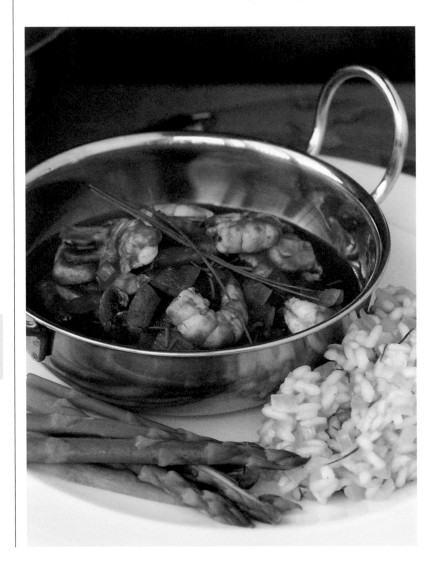

Prawn couscous

1 Pour the vegetable stock into a saucepan, and add the sun-dried tomatoes to soften them.
2 In a large mixing bowl, combine all the vegetables. Sprinkle the couscous over, stir in the herbs and pour in the stock.
3 Cover with a lid for 1 minute to allow the couscous to steam. Remove the lid and fluff up the grains with 2 forks. Mix in the prawns and lemon juice, then transfer to a serving bowl and season with black pepper. Serve with mixed salad leaves.

SERVES 4
PER SERVING
222 CALORIES
4.2G FAT

PREPARATION TIME 10 MINUTES
COOKING TIME 10 MINUTES

420ml hot vegetable stock
4 sun-dried tomatoes (not the type in oil), cut into strips
1 red onion, finely chopped
1 orange and 1 yellow pepper, deseeded and diced
2 small courgettes, diced
100g chestnut mushrooms, sliced
1 tablespoon mixed herbs (e.g. parsley, chives, mint)
175g (dry weight) couscous
200g cooked, shelled prawns
juice of ½ lemon
freshly ground black pepper

TIP *This also tastes good cold as a salad in its own right*

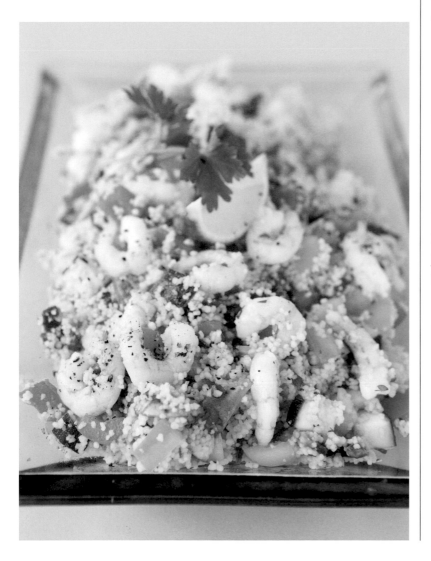

Sage polenta with chilli tomatoes

SERVES 4
PER SERVING
236 CALORIES
3.1G FAT

PREPARATION TIME 20 MINUTES
COOKING TIME 50 MINUTES

225g bramata polenta flour
1.2 litres vegetable stock
1 tablespoon chopped fresh
    sage
1 red onion, finely chopped
2 garlic cloves, crushed
300g cherry tomatoes
1 small red chilli, finely chopped
salt and freshly ground black
    pepper
fresh sage to serve

TIP *Polenta is the flour
derived from maize, or
sweetcorn as we know it. Once
made into a dough, it can be
frozen in squares and reheated
from frozen*

1 Put the polenta flour into a large jug.
2 Pour the vegetable stock into a large saucepan, add the sage and bring to the boil.
3 Slowly whisk the polenta into the stock then, using a wooden spoon, beat well until smooth. Reduce the heat and allow to simmer very gently for 40 minutes to allow the starches to cook out. After 40 minutes the polenta will become a thick paste and start to leave the sides of the pan. Pour into a damp tea towel, and cover while you prepare the chilli tomatoes.
4 Heat a non-stick frying pan, and dry-fry the onion with the remaining garlic until soft and lightly browned. Add the tomatoes and chilli and heat through.
5 Cut the polenta into slices and transfer to a serving plate. Spoon the tomatoes over the polenta and serve with salad.

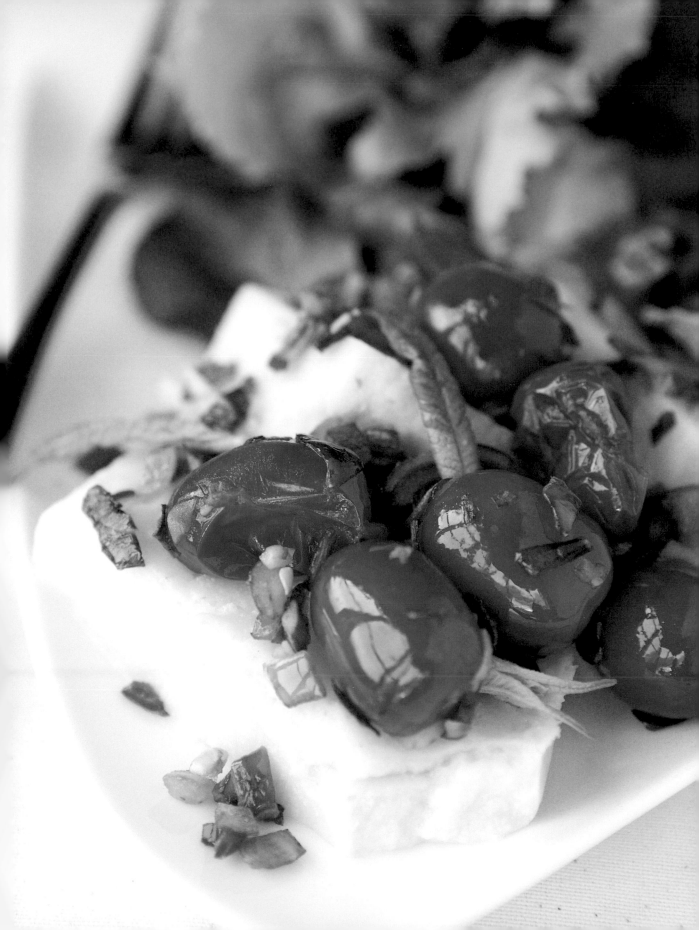

Spicy bean corn rolls

SERVES 4
PER SERVING
172 CALORIES
0.9G FAT

PREPARATION TIME 5 MINUTES

1 x 270g can mixed bean salad,
    drained
1–2 teaspoons chilli sauce
1 tablespoon chopped fresh
    parsley
2 tablespoons low-fat natural
    yogurt
4 corn tortillas
salt and freshly ground black
    pepper

TIP *Spreading the inside of
the tortillas with yogurt helps
to bind the filling together*

1 Place the drained beans in a bowl
  and mix in the chilli sauce and
  chopped parsley.
2 Spread the yogurt over the base of
  the tortillas and season with salt
  and black pepper.
3 Spread the bean mixture over the
  yogurt and roll up the tortillas as
  tightly as possible. Cut each tortilla
  in half and trim the ends.

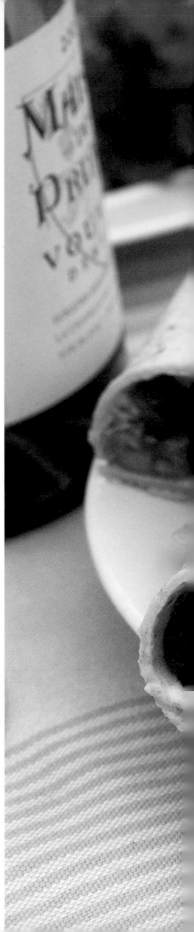

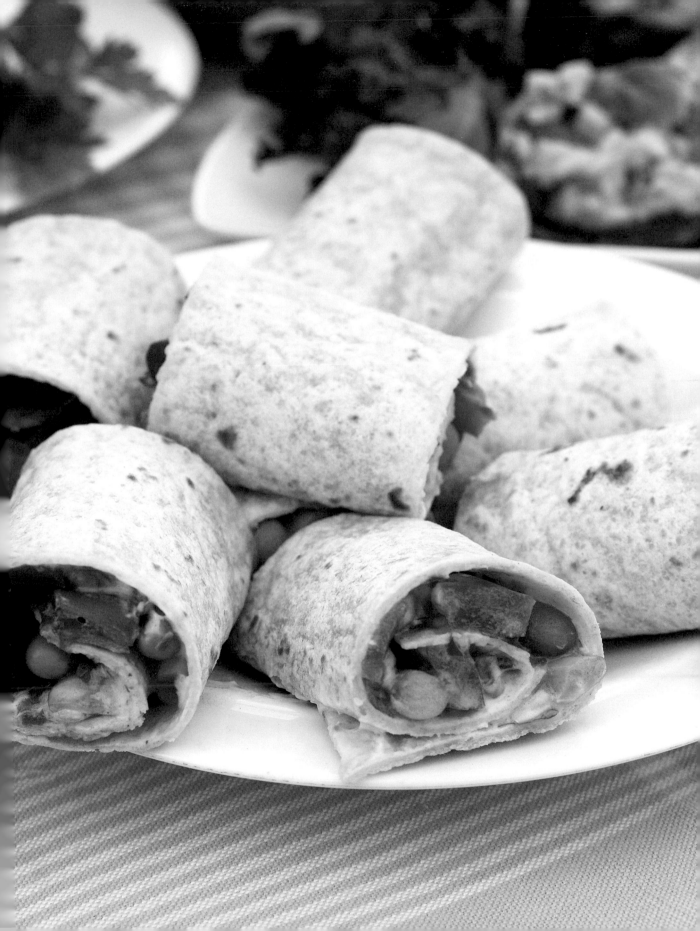

Piri piri chicken

SERVES 4
PER SERVING
236 CALORIES
5.8G FAT

PREPARATION TIME 10 MINUTES
COOKING TIME 20 MINUTES

1 red onion, diced
4 × 175g skinless chicken
    breasts, diced
1 teaspoon ground coriander
1 teaspoon Schwartz pilau rice
    seasoning
1 teaspoon sesame seeds
1 teaspoon vegetable stock
    powder
1 teaspoon cracked black
    pepper

for serving
juice of 1 lemon
4 tablespoons 3 % fat Greek
    yogurt

TIP *Adding fresh lemon to the hot pan adds a really zingy flavour to the chicken*

1 Heat a non-stick wok, and dry-fry the onion until soft. Add the chicken breasts and cook until slightly coloured.
2 Add the remaining ingredients and toss well to make sure the chicken browns on all sides.
3 When the chicken is cooked through, add the lemon juice. Remove from the heat and stir in the yogurt. Serve with mixed salad leaves.

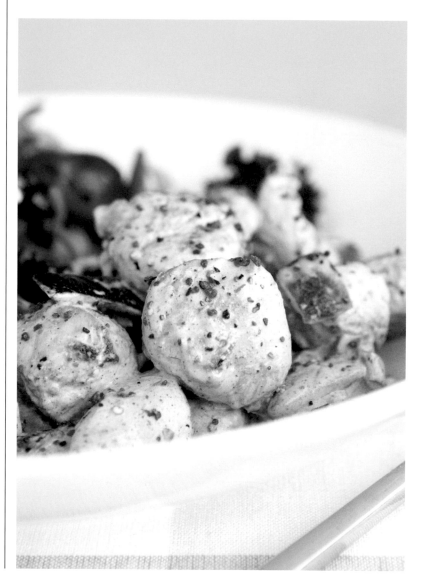

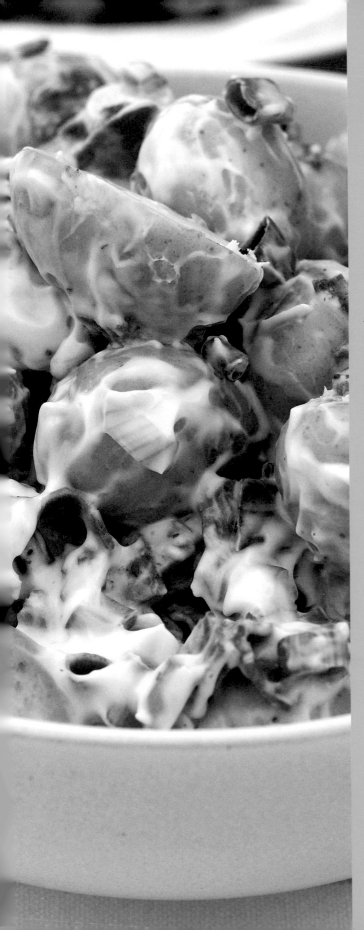

Super salads

This scrumptious selection of salads can be served as lunches, each accompanied by a slice of wholegrain bread or a low-fat yogurt or a piece of fruit, according to your calorie allowance. Alternatively, you can make them up as side salads to accompany supper or dinner party dishes.

Warm chicken Caesar salad

SERVES 4
PER SERVING
167 CALORIES
4.9G FAT

PREPARATION TIME 10 MINUTES
COOKING TIME 10 MINUTES

4 × 120g skinless chicken
   breasts
1 romaine or crisp lettuce
8 spring onions, sliced
½ cucumber

for the dressing
2 tablespoons 2% fat Greek
   yogurt
1 tablespoon low-fat salad
   dressing
1 garlic clove, crushed
fresh lemon juice to taste
salt and freshly ground black
   pepper

TIP *Keep the lettuce in the refrigerator until the chicken is cooked so it stays really crisp*

1 Place the chicken on a chopping board and slice in half horizontally, to create 2 thin escalopes per breast. Season with salt and black pepper.
2 Heat a non-stick griddle pan, and cook the chicken briskly, turning it regularly, for 8–10 minutes.
3 Shred the lettuce, place in a serving bowl and add the sliced spring onions. Using a vegetable peeler, cut the cucumber into very fine strips and add to the salad.
4 Combine the dressing ingredients in a small bowl, thinning the dressing with a little boiling water if required.
5 Arrange the cooked chicken on the salad and drizzle the dressing over.

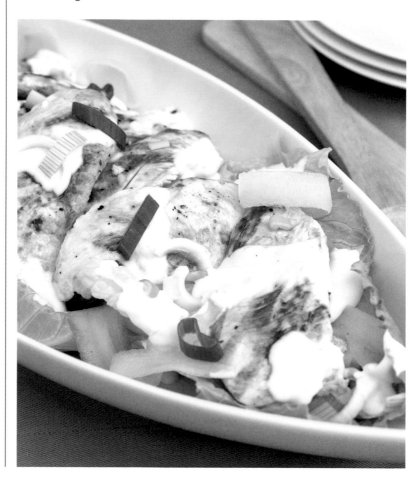

Balsamic bean salad

1 Cook the fine beans and broad beans separately in 2 saucepans of water until tender. Drain and refresh under cold running water.
2 Drain and rinse the canned beans, and place in a bowl. Add the fine beans and broad beans, then the tomatoes, and season with salt and black pepper.
3 Mix together the dressing ingredients and pour over the beans. Toss well, then transfer to a serving dish.

SERVES 4
PER SERVING
187 CALORIES
1.6G FAT

PREPARATION TIME 10 MINUTES
COOKING TIME 10 MINUTES

1 × 200g pack fine green beans
115g baby broad beans
1 × 240g can pinto beans
1 × 175g can cannellini beans
4 tomatoes, skinned and diced
salt and freshly ground black
    pepper

for the dressing
2 tablespoons cloudy apple
    juice
1 tablespoon balsamic vinegar
1 teaspoon grainy mustard

TIP *This salad will keep for 3–4 days in the refrigerator*

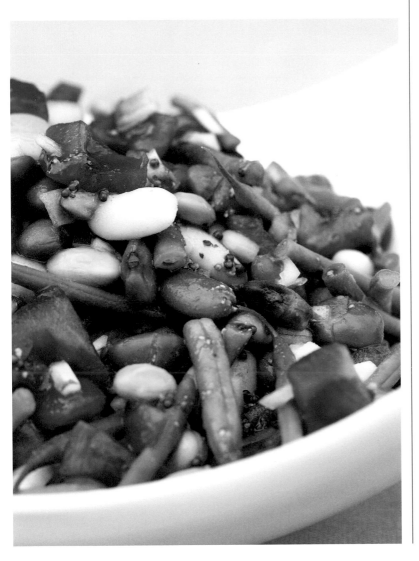

Garlicky Greek salad

SERVES 4
PER SERVING
99 CALORIES
2.9G FAT

PREPARATION TIME 15 MINUTES

1 crisp lettuce
1 cucumber, diced
16 cherry tomatoes, halved
1 red onion, diced
1 red pepper, deseeded and
    diced
75g 50% less fat Le Roule garlic
    and herb cheese
12 black seedless grapes, halved

for the dressing
150ml cloudy apple juice
2 tablespoons white wine
    vinegar
1–2 teaspoons Dijon mustard
1 tablespoon chopped fresh
    parsley
salt and freshly ground black
    pepper

TIP *For a variation, roast the red pepper in the oven and allow to cool before adding to the salad*

1 Shred the lettuce and place in a large serving bowl. Add the cucumber, tomatoes, onion and red pepper.
2 Cut the cheese into small pieces and scatter on the salad along with the grapes.
3 Mix together the dressing ingredients in a bowl and pour over the salad.

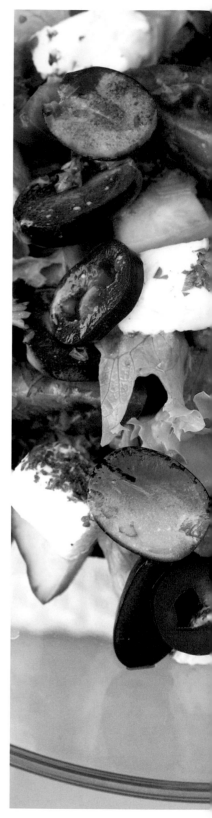

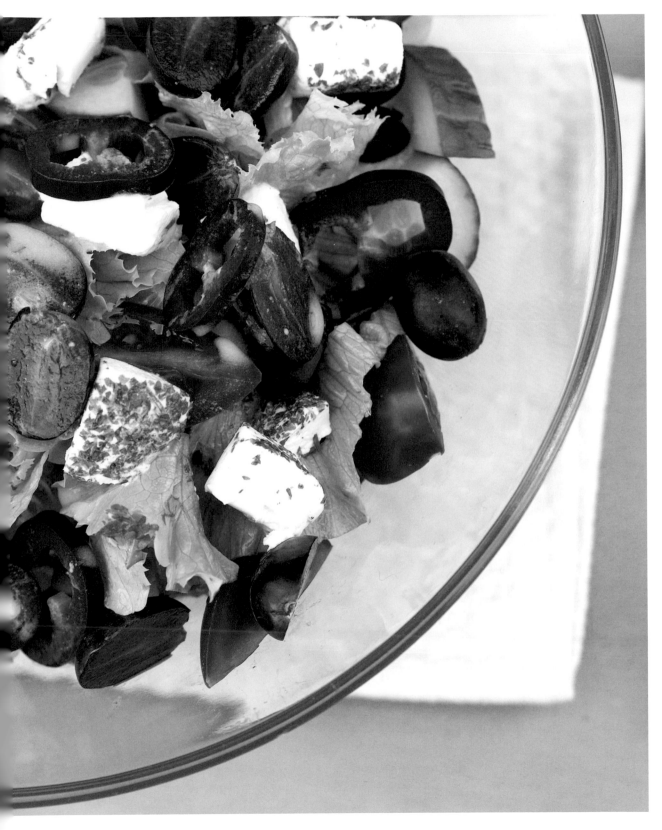

Mango Waldorf salad

SERVES 4
PER SERVING
111 CALORIES
4.2G FAT

PREPARATION TIME 20 MINUTES

1 red eating apple
juice of 1 lemon
1 ripe mango
2 large salad onions, sliced
8 celery sticks, chopped
115g green seedless grapes,
    halved
2 tablespoons 0% fat Greek
    yogurt
1 tablespoon low-fat salad
    cream
1 tablespoon dried cranberries
½ tablespoon pumpkin seeds
salt and freshly ground black
    pepper

TIP *You can leave out the
pumpkin seeds to reduce the
calories and fat even more*

1 Cut the apple into quarters, then cut away the core and discard. Chop the flesh into small pieces and place in a mixing bowl. Add the lemon juice and toss well to coat.
2 Peel the mango, cut the flesh away from the centre stone, then chop it into the bowl. Add the onions, celery and grapes and mix well.
3 Mix together the yogurt and salad cream and add to the salad. Season to taste with salt and black pepper.
4 Spoon into a serving dish, and sprinkle the dried cranberries and pumpkin seeds over the top.

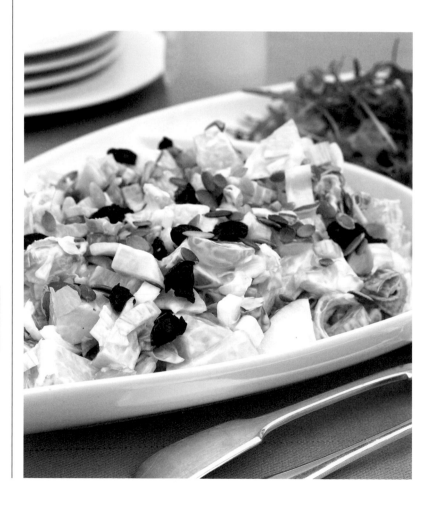

Niçoise-style beef salad

1 Cook the beans in boiling salted water until tender, then drain and refresh under cold running water.
2 Put the refreshed beans in a serving dish and add the potatoes. Cut the tomatoes in half and add to the dish.
3 Heat a non-stick griddle pan. Season the steaks and cook briskly on both sides for 6–8 minutes, depending on the thickness. Remove from the pan and allow to rest.
4 To make the dressing, add the onion to the pan and dry-fry until soft. Add the balsamic vinegar and apple juice and continue to cook until the liquid has reduced by half. Mix in the mustard.
5 Slice the beef into strips and arrange on top of the salad. Drizzle the hot dressing over and serve.

SERVES 4
PER SERVING
268 CALORIES
7.8G FAT

PREPARATION TIME 20 MINUTES
COOKING TIME 15 MINUTES

115g fine green beans
450g small new potatoes, cooked and sliced
20 cherry tomatoes
2 fillet steaks

for the dressing
1 red onion, finely sliced
2 tablespoons balsamic vinegar
2 tablespoons cloudy apple juice
1 teaspoon Dijon mustard
salt and freshly ground black pepper

TIP *If you want, you can use horseradish instead of mustard*

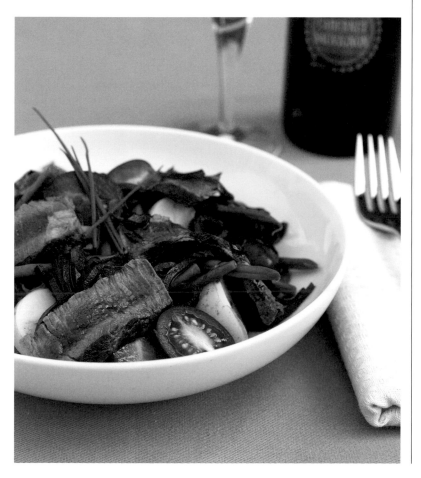

Potato and pastrami salad

SERVES 4
PER SERVING
85 CALORIES
1G FAT

PREPARATION TIME 5 MINUTES
COOKING TIME 20 MINUTES

350g baby potatoes
40g pastrami
juice of ½ lemon
1½ tablespoons extra light
    mayonnaise
salt and freshly ground black
    pepper

TIP *For extra flavour, add a vegetable stock cube and fresh mint to the potato cooking water*

1 Cook the potatoes in a pan of boiling water. Drain and allow to cool.
2 Chop the pastrami into thin strips and add to the cooled potatoes.
3 Mix together the lemon juice and mayonnaise. Spoon over the potatoes, mix well and season to taste with salt and black pepper.

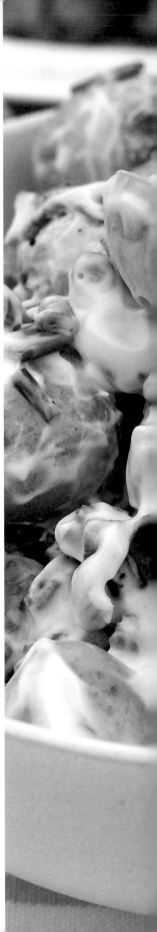

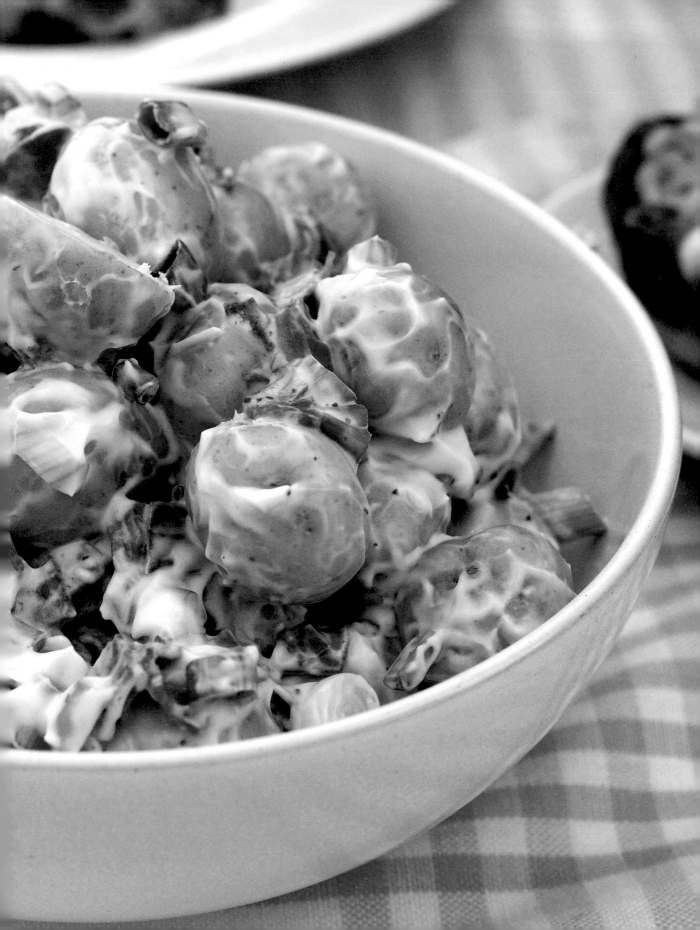

Tomato, mozzarella and red grapefruit salad

SERVES 4
PER SERVING
93 CALORIES
3.6G FAT

PREPARATION TIME 10 MINUTES

4 ripe tomatoes
1 × 125g half-fat mozzarella
1 red grapefruit
salt and freshly ground black
    pepper
fresh basil to garnish

for the dressing
2 tablespoons cloudy apple
    juice
1 tablespoon cider vinegar
1 teaspoon Dijon mustard

TIP *The tomatoes need to be
really ripe to complement the
other ingredients in the salad*

1 Slice the tomatoes and cut the mozzarella into 16 thin slices.
2 Cut away the pith from the grapefruit and cut the grapefruit
into segments, squeezing the juice into a small bowl.
4 Arrange the fruits and cheese on serving plates and season with
salt and black pepper.
5 Mix together the dressing ingredients and the reserved
grapefruit juice. Drizzle on the salad and garnish with fresh basil.

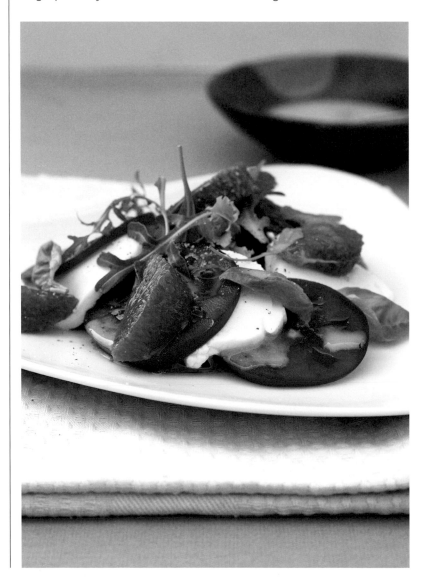

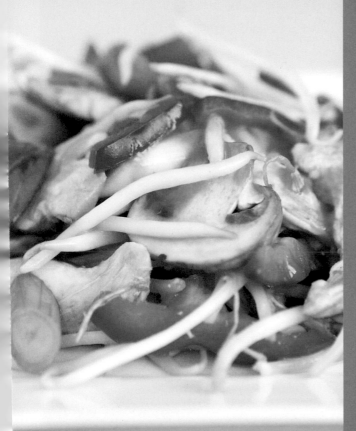

Speedy stir-fries

Stir-fries make fast food healthy and all these recipes can be prepared in 30 minutes or less. The Chilli Beef and Spicy Vegetable Noodle options are good for quick dinners while the others are suitable for lunch or dinner, served with appropriate accompaniments.

Fruity turkey stir-fry

PER SERVING
SERVES 4
233 CALORIES
2.1G FAT

PREPARATION TIME 10 MINUTES
COOKING TIME 10 MINUTES

4 × 120g lean turkey steaks
2 teaspoons ground coriander
1 red onion, finely chopped
2 garlic cloves, crushed
1 × 4cm piece lemongrass,
    finely chopped
1 small red chilli, sliced
300g tomato passata
1 tablespoon chopped fresh
    coriander
2 tablespoons mango chutney
salt and freshly ground black
    pepper

TIP *Coating the turkey with
ground coriander adds a sweet
flavour to the finished dish*

1 Remove any remaining visible fat from the turkey. Slice the steaks into thin strips and place in a shallow dish. Season with salt and black pepper and coat with the ground coriander.

2 Heat a non-stick wok, and dry-fry the onion and garlic until soft. Add the coated turkey strips and cook quickly over a high heat.

3 Add the lemongrass and chilli and toss the ingredients well together. Add the tomato passata and heat through. Remove from the heat, and stir in the fresh coriander and mango chutney. Serve on a bed of boiled basmati rice.

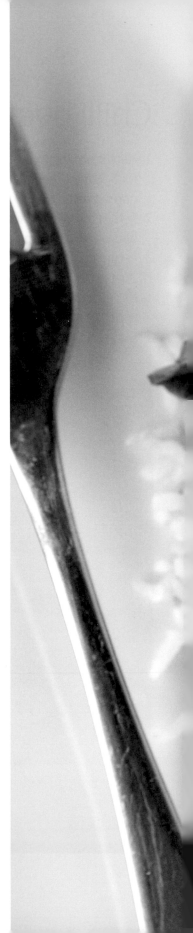

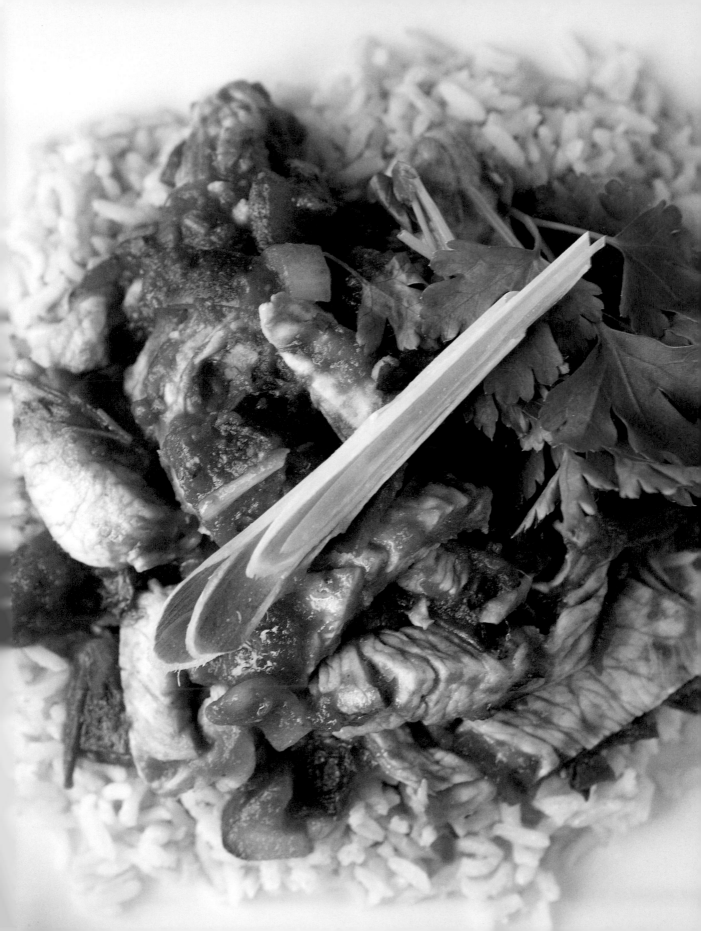

Stir-fry beef with red wine

SERVES 4
PER SERVING
190 CALORIES
5.4G FAT

PREPARATION TIME 10 MINUTES
COOKING TIME 15 MINUTES

4 lean rump steaks, 450g total
1 red onion, finely chopped
2 garlic cloves, crushed
125ml red wine
250g chestnut mushrooms,
    sliced
300ml water
1 teaspoon gravy powder
salt and freshly ground black
    pepper

TIP *Cooking the steaks in a very hot pan seals in the flavour*

1 Remove all visible fat from the meat and season with salt and black pepper.
2 Heat a non-stick frying pan, and seal the meat on both sides, then remove the steaks from the pan and let them rest but keep warm.
3 Add the chopped onion and garlic to the pan and cook until softened soften, then deglaze the pan with the red wine and cook until the wine is reduced by half. Stir in the mushrooms and water.
4 Mix the gravy powder to a paste with a little extra cold water and add to the pan. Return the steaks to the pan and heat through before serving.

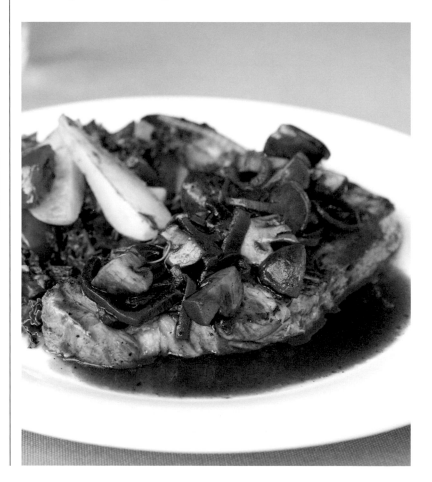

Beef and broccoli stir-fry

1 Mix together the chilli sauce, soy sauce and ginger in a bowl. Add the beef strips and toss well to coat.
2 Heat a non-stick wok, and lightly brown the onion. Add the broccoli florets, mushrooms and coated beef strips. Cook over a high heat until the beef is cooked to your preference.
3 Just before serving, add the beansprouts and black pepper.

SERVES 4
PER SERVING
160 CALORIES
4G FAT

PREPARATION TIME 5 MINUTES
COOKING TIME 10 MINUTES

2 tablespoons sweet chilli sauce
2 tablespoons soy sauce
1 teaspoon chopped fresh
    ginger
2 × 125g lean rump steaks, cut
    into strips
1 red onion, chopped
250g small broccoli florets
200g chestnut mushrooms,
    quartered
335g fresh beansprouts
freshly ground black pepper

TIP *Adding the beansprouts just before serving gives a crunchy texture to the stir-fry*

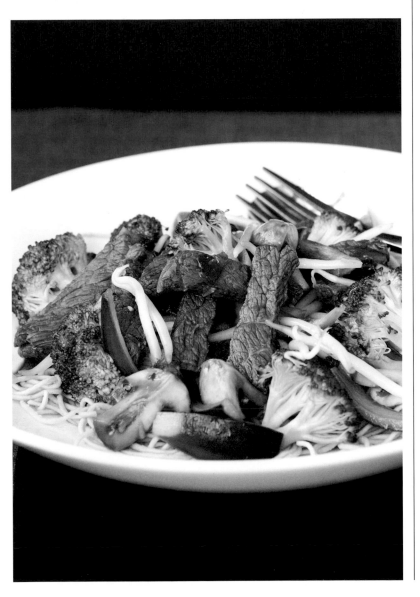

Unbelievably creamy chicken korma with rice

SERVES 4
PER SERVING
415 CALORIES
5.6G FAT

PREPARATION TIME 10 MINUTES
COOKING TIME 20 MINUTES

200g (dry weight) basmati rice
3 × 150g skinless chicken
    breasts, sliced
1 red onion, chopped
2 garlic cloves, crushed
2–3 teaspoons curry powder
150ml vegetable stock
1 tablespoon plain flour
300ml semi-skimmed milk
2 tablespoons low-fat yogurt
1 tablespoon chopped fresh
    coriander to garnish
salad leaves to serve

TIP *Remember not to add the yogurt until the wok is off the heat as it will curdle if boiled*

1 Preheat a non-stick wok. Put the rice in a pan of boiling water to cook while you prepare the chicken.
2 Add the chicken to the hot wok and lightly brown on all sides.
3 Add the onion and garlic and stir in the curry powder, and cook until the onion is brown.
4 Add 2 tablespoons of the vegetable stock, then stir in the flour and cook out for 1 minute before gradually stirring in the milk and the remaining stock. Simmer for 10 minutes, then remove from the heat and stir in the yogurt.
5 Drain the rice and arrange on serving plates.
6 Sprinkle the coriander over the chicken and spoon on to the rice. Serve with salad leaves.

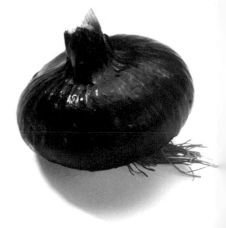

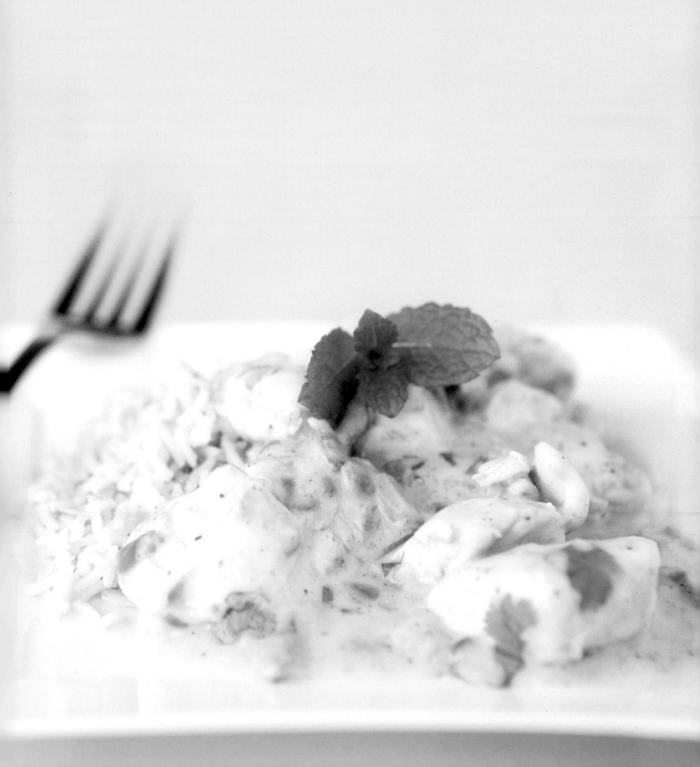

Gammon with creamy wild mushrooms

SERVES 4
PER SERVING
193 KCAL
9.3G FAT

PREPARATION TIME 5 MINUTES
COOKING TIME 20 MINUTES

4 × 120g gammon steaks
60ml white wine
250g mixed mushrooms
4 tablespoons 3% fat Greek
   yogurt
squeeze of lemon juice
1 tbsp chopped fresh parsley
freshly ground black pepper

TIP *Gammon is a good standby – store in the freezer and defrost in a bowl of water*

1 Heat a non-stick griddle pan, and cook the gammon steaks quickly on both sides. Remove from the pan and keep warm.
2 Deglaze the pan with the white wine and cook until the mixture is reduced by half. Stir in the mushrooms and cook until soft. Remove the pan from the heat and stir in the yogurt. Add the lemon juice and black pepper to taste. Stir in the parsley and serve.
3 Serve the gammon steaks with the creamy mushroom sauce.

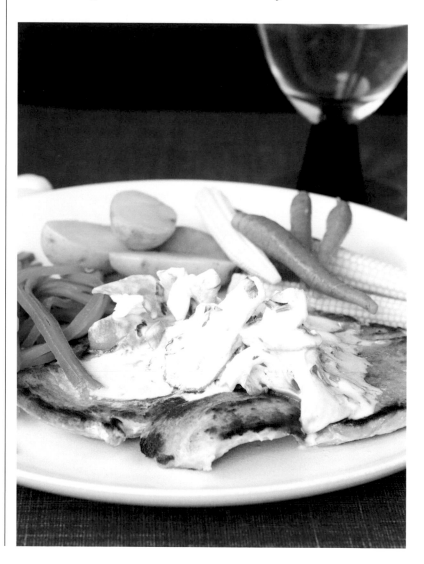

Spicy vegetable noodle stir-fry

1 Heat a non-stick wok or frying pan, and dry-fry the spring onions, courgettes, red and yellow peppers and fresh ginger until lightly coloured.
2 Add the sliced chilli and cook for a further 2–3 minutes. Stir in the remaining ingredients. Add the noodles, mix well and heat through. Serve immediately.

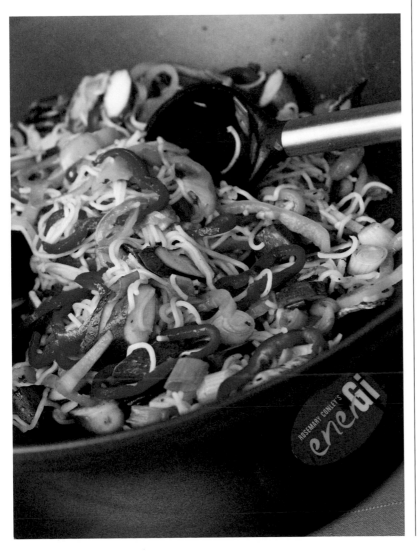

PER SERVING
SERVES 4
390 CALORIES
5.8G FAT

PREPARATION TIME 10 MINUTES
COOKING TIME 10 MINUTES

8 spring onions, finely sliced
4 baby courgettes, sliced
1 red pepper, deseeded and
    finely sliced
1 yellow pepper, deseeded and
    finely sliced
1 × 2cm piece fresh ginger,
    peeled and finely chopped
1 small red chilli, sliced
4–5 chestnut mushrooms, sliced
1 teaspoon light soy sauce
1 teaspoon Bengal spice mango
    chutney
1 teaspoon runny honey
juice of 1 lemon
1 × 150g pack straight to wok
    fine noodles

TIP *For a slight variation substitute 1–2 teaspoons lime pickle for the soy sauce*

Vegetable and black bean noodle stir-fry

SERVES 4
PER SERVING
199 CALORIES
3G FAT

PREPARATION TIME 10 MINUTES
COOKING TIME 10 MINUTES

2 red onions, finely sliced
2 garlic cloves, crushed
1 green and 1 red pepper,
   deseeded
1 × 100g pack baby asparagus
1 × 100g pack ready to wok Pad
   Thai noodles
1 × 125g pack baby corn
150ml black bean sauce
2 tablespoons low-salt soy
   sauce
1 tablespoon runny honey
zest and juice of 1 lime
freshly ground black pepper

TIP *For a fresh herb flavour,
add some chopped fresh
coriander to your noodles as
you drain them*

1 Heat a non-stick wok, and dry-fry the onions and garlic for 3–4
   minutes over a high heat, seasoning well with black pepper.
2 Slice the peppers and add to the wok along with the asparagus,
   and cook for a further 1–2 minutes.
3 Add the noodles and the remaining ingredients and toss well
   together for 3–4 minutes. Serve straight away.

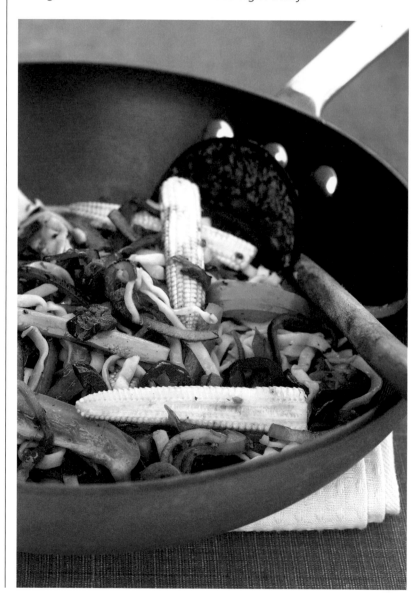

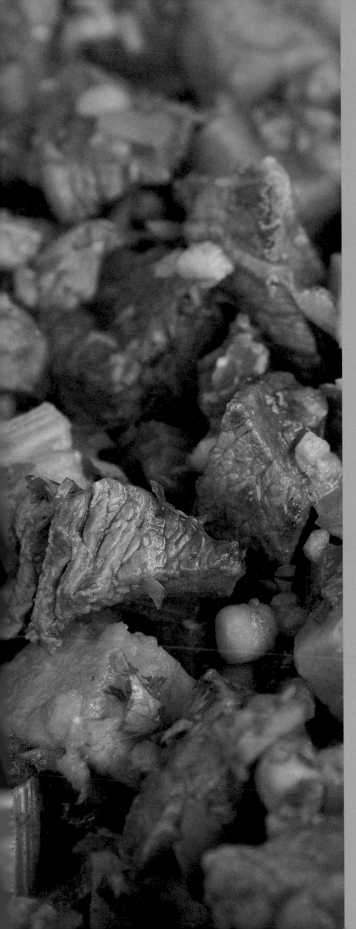

Casseroles and curries

Most of these dishes are best made in advance on a long, slow simmer so that the flavours have plenty of time to imbue, which improves the taste. Many are suitable for freezing, ready to be thawed out and then reheated for an easy dinner or supper option on busy days.

Pork and chickpea casserole

SERVES 4
PER SERVING
320 CALORIES
7.6G FAT

PREPARATION TIME 10 MINUTES
COOKING TIME 45 MINUTES

1 red onion, cut into wedges
2 garlic cloves, finely chopped
4 × 100g lean pork slices
1 teaspoon ground coriander
1 teaspoon ground cumin
2 x 400g cans chopped
    tomatoes
2 teaspoons vegetable bouillon
    stock powder
2 tablespoons dry sherry
1 × 400g can chickpeas
1 tablespoon chopped fresh
    thyme
zest and juice of 1 orange
1 tablespoon chopped fresh
    parsley

TIP *If you don't have a lid that fits your dish, cover with foil and scrunch up around the sides for a tight fit*

1 Preheat the oven to 180C, 350F, gas mark 4.
2 Heat a heavy-based, non-stick pan, and dry-fry the onion and garlic until soft. Transfer to an ovenproof dish or casserole.
3 Season the pork on both sides with black pepper, then add to the non-stick pan and brown them on both sides. Sprinkle with the spices and transfer to the dish.
4 Add the chopped tomatoes, stock powder, sherry and chickpeas to the pan. Reduce the heat and simmer for 2–3 minutes, adding the orange zest, juice and the thyme as the sauce thickens.
5 Pour the sauce over the pork, cover with a lid, and place in the oven for 30 minutes until cooked through.
6 Transfer to a serving dish and sprinkle with chopped parsley.

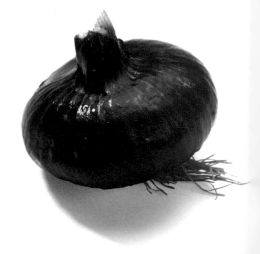

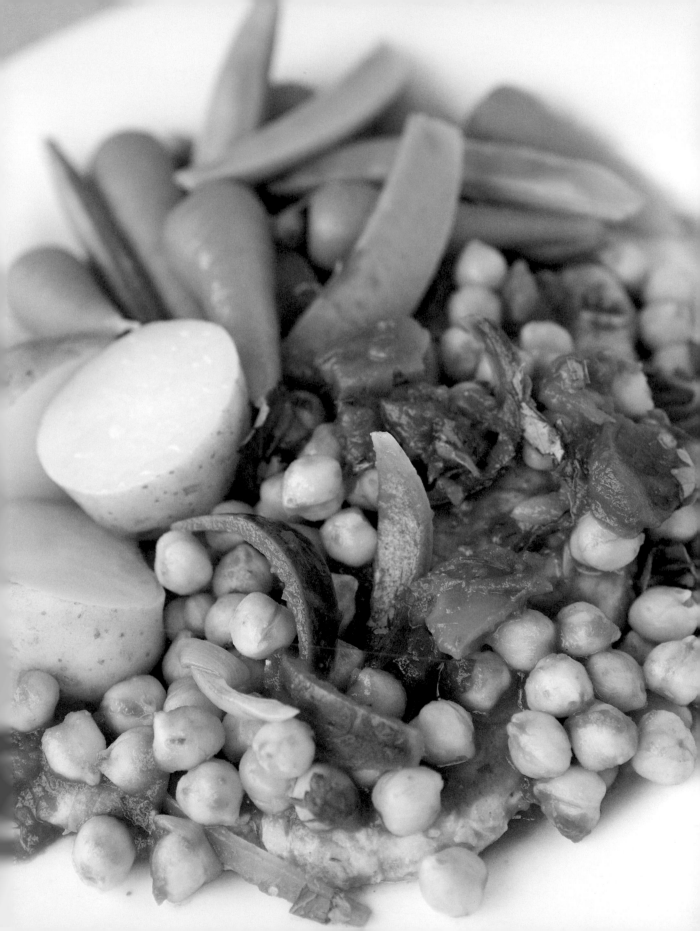

Chicken and pearl barley casserole

SERVES 4
PER SERVING
386 CALORIES
6.2G FAT

PREPARATION TIME 15 MINUTES
COOKING TIME 1 HOUR

2 medium onions, diced
2 garlic cloves, crushed
4 × 160g skinless chicken
    breasts
100g soup mix with dried pulses
    (e.g. Goodness)
4 carrots, diced
1 large turnip, diced
2 celery sticks, chopped
1 litre chicken stock
1 tablespoon chopped fresh
    thyme
450g potatoes, peeled and
    diced
freshly ground black pepper
2 tablespoons chopped fresh
    parsley to garnish

TIP *You can also cook this
dish in a slow cooker or electric
wok over a low heat*

1 Heat a non-stick frying pan, and dry-fry the onions and garlic for
   2–3 minutes until soft.
2 Add the chicken breasts, season with black pepper, and
   continue to cook over a high heat until well sealed.
3 Transfer to a large casserole pan and add the vegetables,
   chicken stock and thyme.
4 Rinse the soup mix with pulses well and add to the pan along
   with the potatoes. Cover and simmer gently for 1 hour.
5 Sprinkle the parsley over and serve.

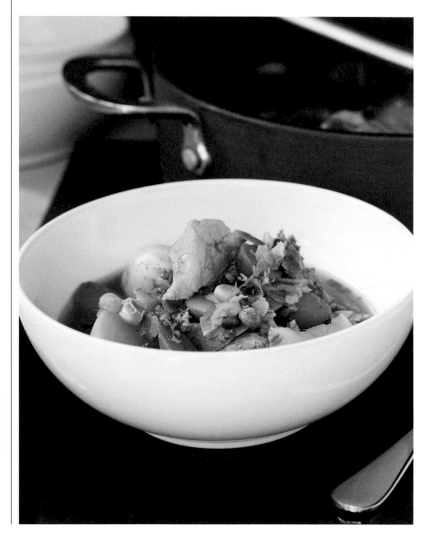

Beef pasanda

1 Heat a non-stick frying pan, and dry-fry the onion and garlic until the onion is lightly browned. Add the beef and cook until sealed, then season with black pepper.
2 Add the ginger, ground coriander and curry powder, then cook, mixing well, before adding the stock cube and canned tomatoes.
3 Cover and simmer for 30–35 minutes until the beef is tender and the sauce reduced.
4 Sprinkle the coriander over and serve.

SERVES 4
PER SERVING
202 CALORIES
6.4G FAT

PREPARATION TIME 10 MINUTES
COOKING TIME 35 MINUTES

1 red onion, diced
2 garlic cloves, crushed
450g lean frying steak, sliced
1 × 2cm piece fresh ginger, peeled and finely chopped
2 teaspoons ground coriander
1 tablespoon medium curry powder
1 beef stock cube
2 × 400g cans chopped tomatoes
freshly ground black pepper
fresh coriander to serve

TIP *Make sure you cook out the spices so you end up with a mellow-flavoured curry*

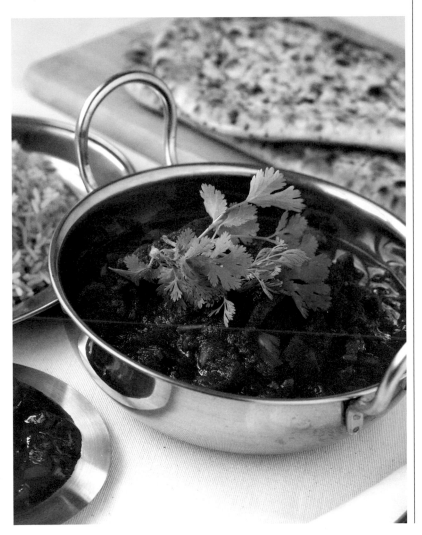

Hearty beef casserole

PER SERVING
SERVES 4
377 CALORIES
6.9G FAT

PREPARATION TIME 15 MINUTES
COOKING TIME 1 HOUR 10 MINUTES

2 medium onions, diced
2 garlic cloves, crushed
450g lean diced beef
4 carrots, diced
450g sweet potato, peeled and
    diced
2 celery sticks, chopped
1 litre meat stock
2 tablespoons tomato purée
bouquet garni
100g country soup mix (pulses,
    peas and barley)
freshly ground black pepper
2 tablespoons chopped fresh
    parsley to garnish

TIP *A good recipe to make in a slow cooker a day in advance*

1 Heat a heavy-based, non-stick pan, and dry-fry the onion and garlic for 2–3 minutes until soft.
2 Add the beef, season well with black pepper, and continue to cook over a high heat until well sealed.
3 Transfer to a large casserole, then add the vegetables, meat stock, tomato purée and bouquet garni. Rinse the pulses well and add to the pan. Cover and simmer gently for 1 hour or until the meat is tender.
4 Sprinkle with the parsley before serving.

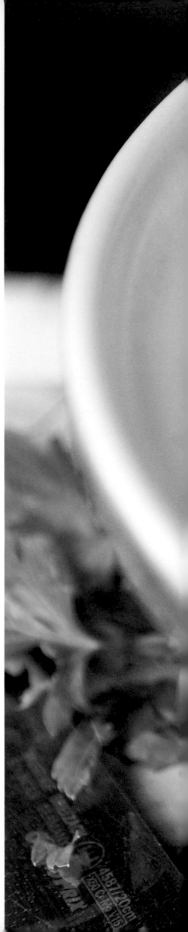

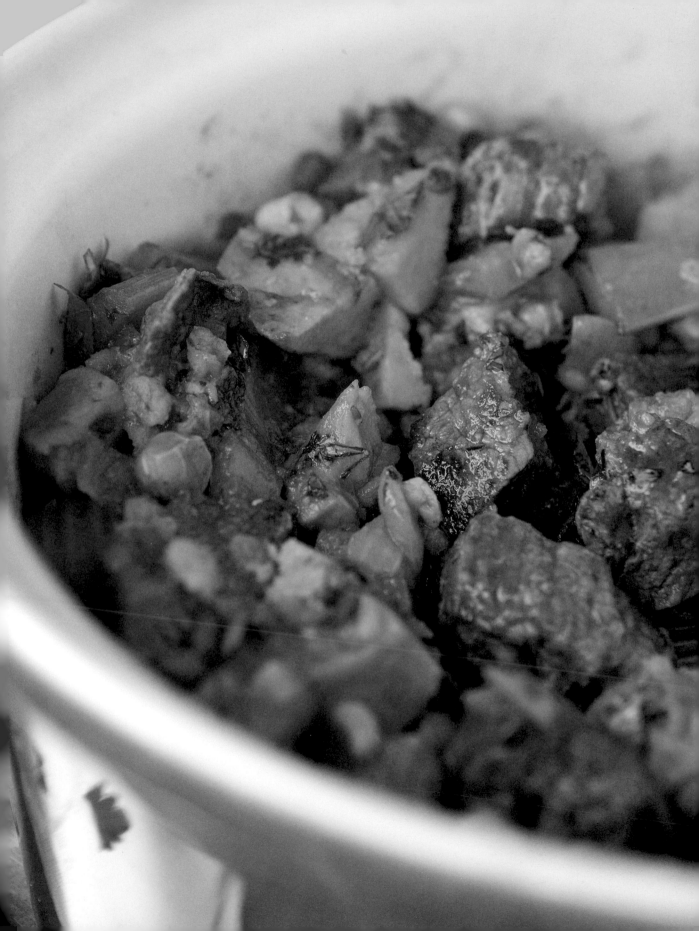

Lamb tagine

SERVES 4
PER SERVING
251 CALORIES
9.2G FAT

PREPARATION TIME 10 MINUTES
COOKING TIME 45 MINUTES

1 large onion, finely diced
2 garlic cloves, crushed
450g very lean diced lamb
1 teaspoon coriander seeds
1 teaspoon ground cinnamon
½ teaspoon cayenne pepper
seeds from 6 cardamom pods
450ml meat stock
2 tablespoons plain flour
1 tablespoon chopped fresh
    marjoram
1 × 400g can chopped
    tomatoes
1 orange
freshly ground black pepper
fresh mint to garnish

TIP *Cook this dish slowly over a low heat for maximum flavour*

1 Heat a non-stick pan, and dry-fry the onion and garlic until soft. Add the lamb and spices, and continue to cook, sealing the meat on all sides.
2 Add 2 tablespoons of meat stock, then sprinkle with the flour. Cook out the flour for 1 minute before adding the remaining stock, chopped marjoram and tomatoes.
3 Cut the orange into small wedges and add to the pan. Cover with a lid and simmer gently for 45 minutes until the lamb is tender, adding more stock if required. Season with black pepper and garnish with fresh mint.

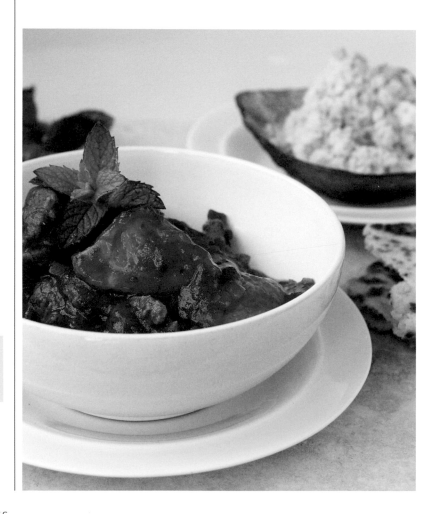

Bombay chicken

1 Preheat the oven to 200C, 400F, gas mark 6.
2 Place the chicken breasts on a chopping board and season on both sides with salt and black pepper. Make an incision to form a pocket in the side of each fillet. Place 2 teaspoons of mango chutney inside each fillet.
3 Put the spices in a bowl and press each chicken breast into them, coating both sides. Transfer to a non-stick baking tray and bake, uncovered, for 25–30 minutes until the chicken is fully cooked. Cut the breasts in half to check they are cooked right through to the centre. Serve on a bed of boiled basmati rice mixed with chopped peppers.

SERVES 4
PER SERVING
243 CALORIES
6.5G FAT

PREPARATION TIME 20 MINUTES
COOKING TIME 30 MINUTES

4 × 175g skinless chicken
    breasts
6 teaspoons mango chutney
2 teaspoons ground turmeric
2 teaspoons ground coriander
2 teaspoons ground ginger
2 teaspoons tandoori powder
salt and freshly ground black
    pepper

TIP *Mix together some chopped fresh coriander and a little low-fat yogurt to make a simple sauce to serve alongside the chicken*

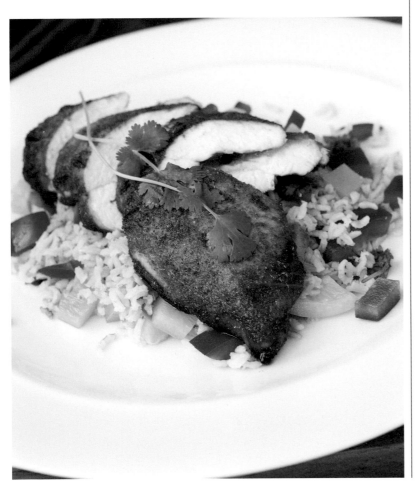

Neil and Allyson's speedy chicken curry

SERVES 4
PER SERVING
224 CALORIES
5.6G FAT

PREPARATION TIME 10 MINUTES
COOKING TIME 20 MINUTES

1 red onion, chopped
1 garlic clove, crushed
1 teaspoon cumin seeds
1 teaspoon ground turmeric
1 teaspoon garam masala
½ teaspoon chilli paste
1 teaspoon ground ginger
4 × 175g skinless chicken
    breasts, cut into chunks
1–2 teaspoons vegetable stock
    powder
1 × 400g can plum tomatoes,
    blended
2 tablespoons 3% fat natural
    yogurt
1 tablespoon chopped fresh
    coriander, plus extra for
    garnishing
freshly ground black pepper

TIP *If freezing this dish, don't add the yogurt until you're ready to serve*

1 Heat a non-stick frying pan, and dry-fry the onion and garlic until soft. Add the spices and cook for 1–2 minutes.
2 Add the chicken chunks and move them round the pan to coat with the spices. Once the chicken has changed colour, add the vegetable stock powder and blended tomatoes, and season with black pepper. Simmer gently for 20 minutes until the chicken is cooked.
3 Just before serving, remove from the heat and stir in the yogurt and chopped coriander. Garnish with fresh coriander.

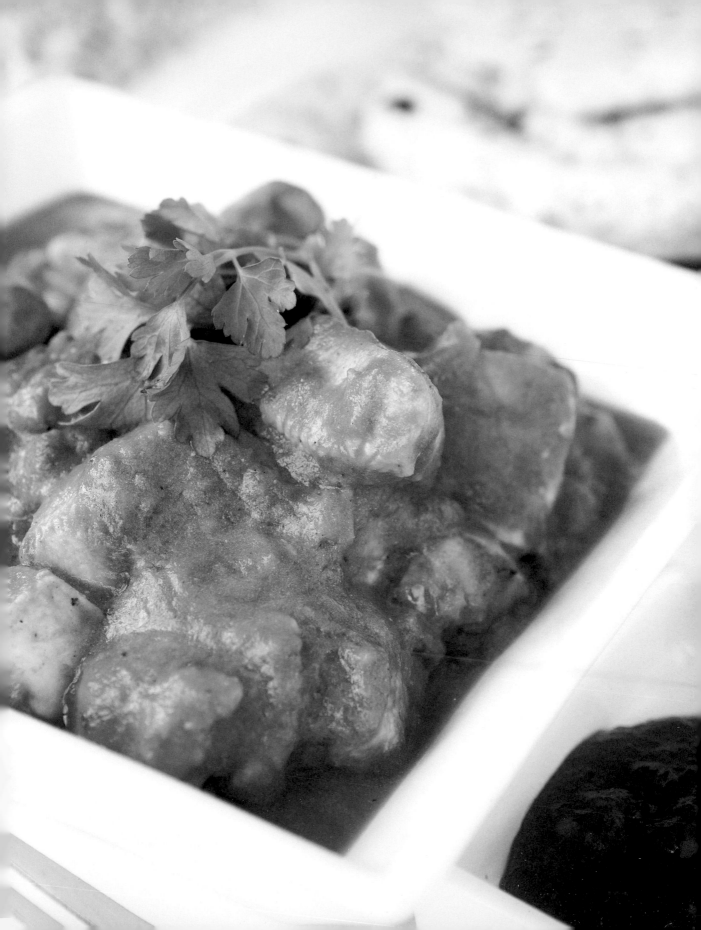

Green Thai chicken curry

SERVES 4
PER SERVING
324 CALORIES
15.2G FAT

PREPARATION TIME 15 MINUTES
COOKING TIME 30 MINUTES

2 onions, diced
2 garlic cloves, chopped
4 × 160g skinless chicken
    breasts, cut into dice
1 tablespoon ground coriander
½ teaspoon ground turmeric
¼ teaspoon fenugreek seeds or
    ground fenugreek
1 small fresh red chilli, chopped
seeds from 4 cardamom pods
4 Kaffir lime leaves (optional)
1–2 teaspoons chicken stock
    powder
1 × 400ml can reduced-fat
    coconut milk
2 tablespoons chopped fresh
    basil
115g shredded fresh spinach
freshly ground black pepper

TIP *Make sure you use
reduced-fat coconut milk,
otherwise you'll be adding
unnecessary fat and calories*

1 Heat a non-stick wok or frying pan, and dry-fry the onions and
  garlic until soft and lightly coloured. Add the chicken and seal
  the outside of the meat. Season with black pepper.
2 Add the spices and cook for a further 2 minutes before adding
  the stock powder and coconut milk.
3 Reduce the heat and allow to simmer gently as the sauce
  thickens.
4 Just before serving, stir in the chopped basil and shredded
  spinach. Serve with boiled basmati rice.

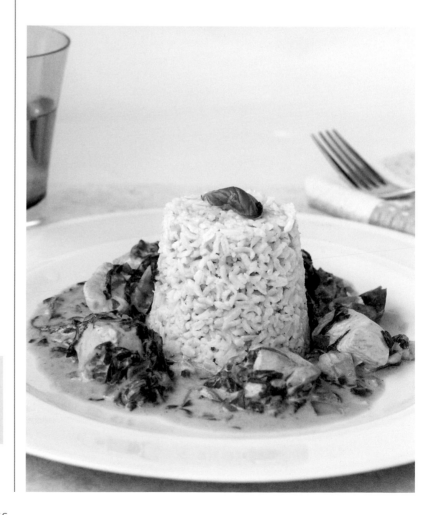

Baked monkfish chermoula

1 Preheat the oven to 200C, 400F, gas mark 6.
2 Using a sharp knife, cut down the centre of each tail removing 2 fillets from each tail. Cut away the skin.
3 Mix together the spices and spread the spice mix on a plate.
4 Roll the fish through the spices and place on a non-stick baking tray. Squeeze the lime juice over the fish and bake in the oven for 10–15 minutes.
5 Remove the fish from the oven and allow to rest for 1 minute. Serve on a bed of wilted spinach with steamed vegetables or salad and boiled new potatoes (with skins). Garnish with lime wedges.

SERVES 4
PER SERVING
90 CALORIES
0.8G FAT

PREPARATION TIME 15 MINUTES
COOKING TIME 15 MINUTES

4 monkfish tails, approx. 130g each
1 teaspoon ground cumin
1 teaspoon paprika
1 teaspoon ground turmeric
pinch of saffron
1 small red chilli, finely chopped
zest and juice of 1 lime
salt and freshly ground black pepper
lime wedges to garnish

TIP *When preparing monkfish, rub it with coarse sea salt. This makes it easier to pull away the skin*

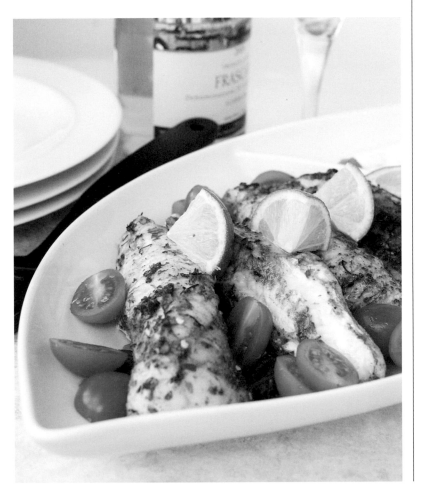

Fragrant fish curry

SERVES 4
PER SERVING
284 CALORIES
3.8G FAT

PREPARATION TIME 10 MINUTES
COOKING TIME 20 MINUTES

1 large red onion, finely
   chopped
1 red pepper, deseeded and
   diced
2 garlic cloves, crushed
1 teaspoon ground coriander
1 teaspoon finely chopped
   lemongrass
1 tablespoon flour
600ml semi-skimmed milk
1–2 teaspoons vegetable stock
   powder
1 small red chilli, finely sliced
1 Kaffir lime leaf
800g fresh boneless cod loin,
   cut into chunks
1 tablespoon chopped fresh
   coriander

TIP *Choose thick, chunky cuts
of fish so they don't fall apart
during cooking*

1 Heat a non-stick wok or frying pan.
Add the onion, red pepper and
garlic and dry-fry for 2–3 minutes
until soft.
2 Stir in the ground coriander and the
lemongrass. Add 1–2 tablespoons
of milk and sprinkle the flour over.
Cook out the flour for 1 minute,
then gradually stir in the remaining
milk and the stock powder.
3 Add the chilli and Kaffir lime leaf
and bring to a gentle simmer. Add
the cod and cook for a further 5
minutes until the sauce has reduced
slightly.
4 Remove from the heat and stir in
the fresh coriander. Serve on a bed
of boiled basmati rice.

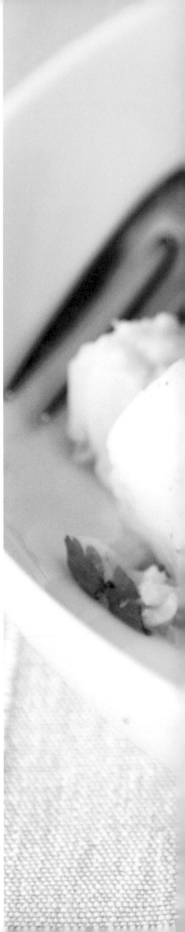

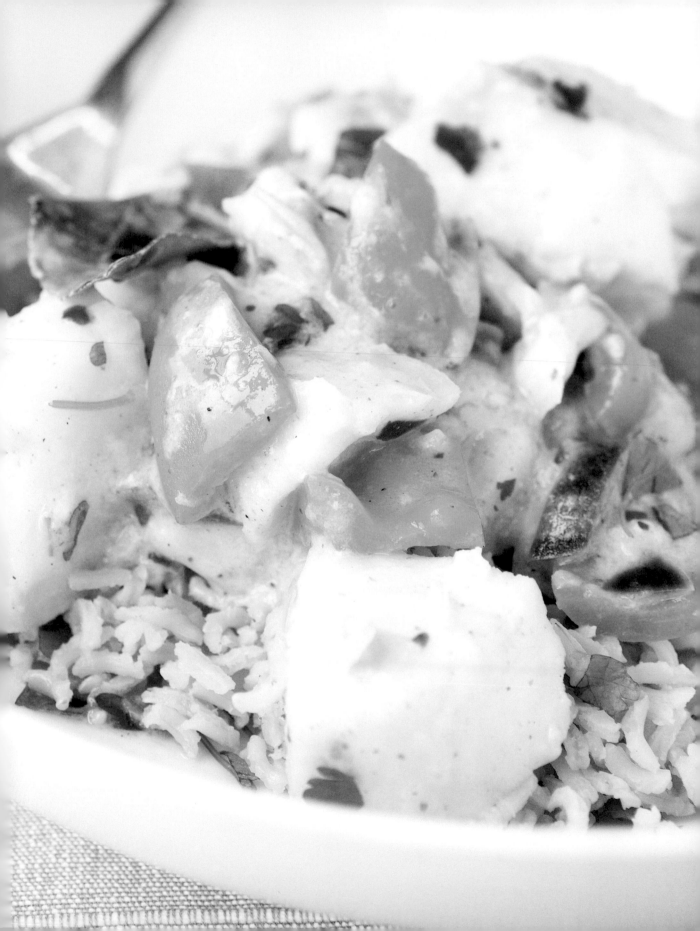

Aubergine green Thai curry

SERVES 4
PER SERVING
194 CALORIES
12.3G FAT

PREPARATION TIME 5 MINUTES
COOKING TIME 30 MINUTES

1 large aubergine, diced
1 red onion, diced
2 garlic cloves, crushed
1 tablespoon green Thai curry
  paste
1 butternut squash, peeled and
  cut into dice
1 × 400ml can reduced-fat
  coconut milk
1 teaspoon vegetable stock
  powder
1 red chilli, chopped
160g fresh peas
basil leaves to garnish

TIP *Always use a serrated knife to cut aubergine as it slices through the skin more easily*

1 Heat a non-stick wok, and dry-fry the aubergine, red onion and garlic for 5–6 minutes.
2 Add the curry paste and the squash and continue cooking for a further 5 minutes.
3 Stir in the coconut milk, stock powder and red chilli. Simmer gently for 15 minutes to allow the squash to soften, adding a little water if required.
4 About 2 minutes before serving, stir in the peas, and heat through. Garnish with basil leaves.

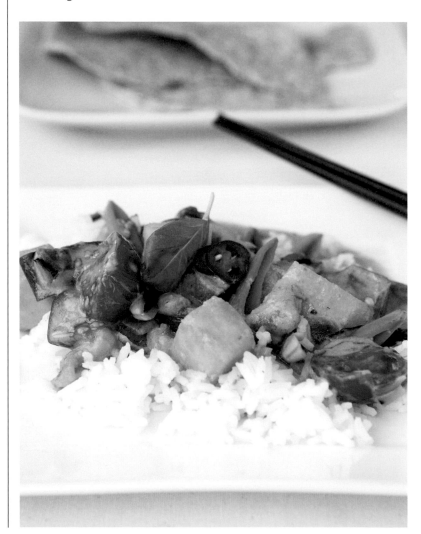

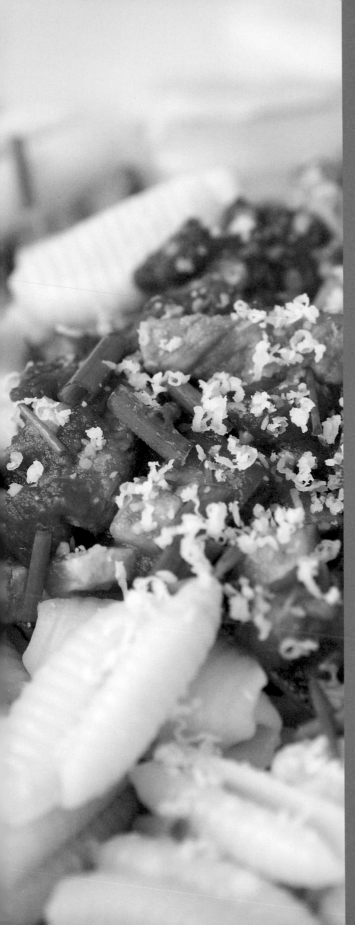

Pasta and pizza

Put some passion into your cooking with these perfect pizza and pasta dishes. They may not be quite like Mamma used to make them, but these low-fat alternatives certainly won't disappoint on taste and they'll do your waistline a big favour too. *Ciao*!

Farfalle bolognese

SERVES 4
PER SERVING
328 CALORIES
7G FAT

PREPARATION TIME 10 MINUTES
COOKING TIME 20 MINUTES

225g (dry weight) farfalle pasta
1 vegetable stock cube
1 red onion, finely chopped
1 garlic clove, crushed
225g lean minced beef
pinch of chilli flakes
2 × 400g cans chopped
    tomatoes
1 tablespoon chopped fresh
    mixed herbs
salt and freshly ground black
    pepper
a few chopped chives to garnish

TIP *Spice up your pasta sauce by mixing a few dried chilli flakes into the sauce*

1 Cook the pasta in a large pan of boiling water with the vegetable stock cube.
2 Heat a non-stick pan, and dry-fry the onion and garlic until soft. Add the beef and cook until it completely changes colour. Add the chilli flakes, tomatoes and mixed herbs, season with salt and black pepper and cook for a further 15–20 minutes until the sauce thickens.
3 Drain the pasta and pour it into a warmed serving dish. Spoon the sauce on top and garnish with chopped chives.

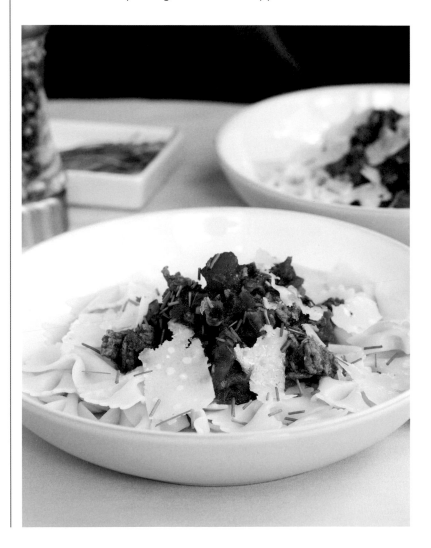

Smoked haddock and corn lasagne

1. Preheat the oven to 200C, 400F, gas mark 6.
2. Skin the smoked haddock and cut into small chunks, checking for bones.
3. Mix 2 tablespoons of milk with the cornflour. Heat the remaining milk in a saucepan, When the milk is hot whisk in the cornflour paste along with the stock powder, mustard, chives and wine. Mix in half the cheese and season with salt and black pepper.
4. Place a thin layer of sauce in the base of an ovenproof dish. Add a layer of pasta sheets then cover with a layer of smoked haddock and sweetcorn. Continue layering, and finish with a top layer of sauce. Sprinkle the remaining cheese on top and place in the oven for 25–30 minutes until golden brown and cooked through.

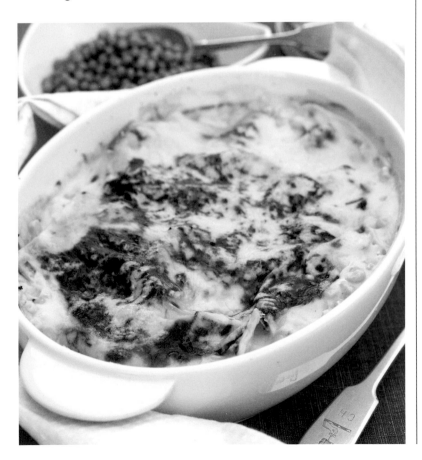

SERVES 4
PER SERVING
431 CALORIES
6.8G FAT

PREPARATION TIME 15 MINUTES
COOKING TIME 40 MINUTES

225g smoked haddock
600ml semi-skimmed milk
2 tablespoons cornflour
1–2 teaspoons vegetable stock powder
2 teaspoons Dijon mustard
1 tablespoon chopped fresh chives
150ml white wine
50g Rosemary Conley mature cheese, grated
225g no pre-cook lasagne sheets
225g frozen sweetcorn, defrosted
salt and freshly ground black pepper

TIP *Try not to have the sauce too thick as it will be absorbed into the pasta as it cooks*

Pancetta and mushroom pasta

PER SERVING
SERVES 4
268 CALORIES
3.8G FAT

PREPARATION TIME 10 MINUTES
COOKING TIME 25 MINUTES

225g (dry weight) pasta shapes
1 vegetable stock cube,
4 × 15g slices pancetta, cut into
  strips
1 small red onion, finely
  chopped,
1 garlic clove, crushed,
225g chestnut mushrooms,
  sliced
2 baby courgettes, finely diced,
pinch of cayenne pepper
1 × 400g can chopped
  tomatoes,
2 tablespoons chopped fresh
  chives

TIP *You can also use this sauce for grilled meat and fish or as a topping for toast or jacket potatoes*

1 Cook the pasta in a large saucepan of boiling water with the stock cube.
2 Heat a non-stick pan, and dry-fry the pancetta, onion and garlic and until soft.
3 Add the mushrooms and courgettes, and continue cooking for 2–3 minutes. Add the remaining ingredients and simmer gently for 5–6 minutes.
4 Drain the pasta thoroughly, arrange on warmed plates and pour the sauce over the top. Garnish with the chives.

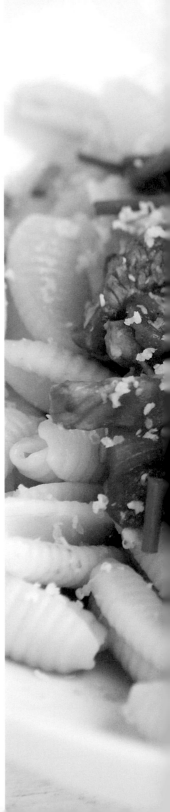

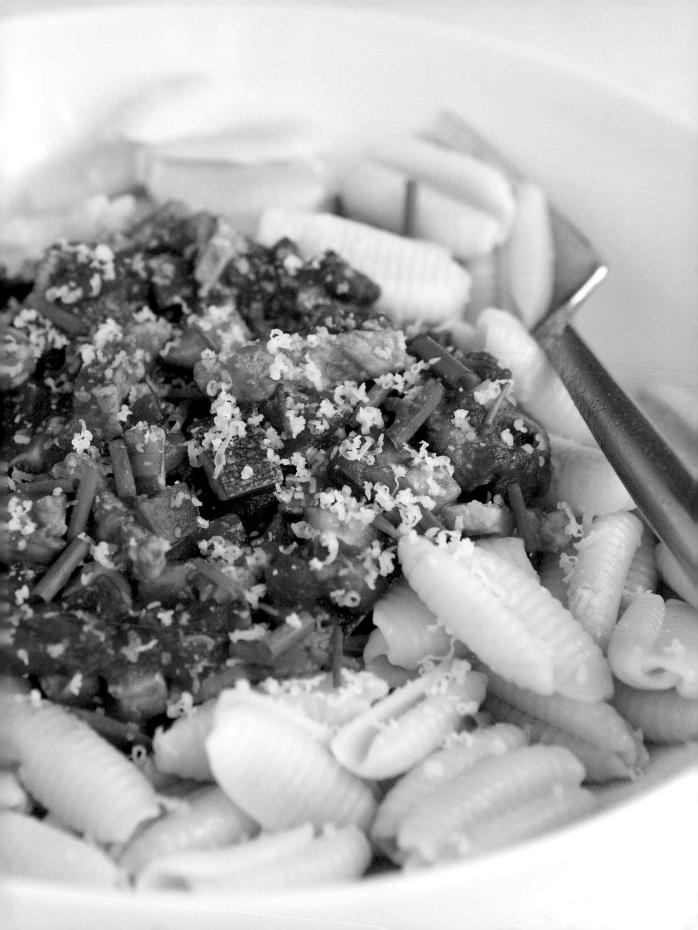

Tagliatelle carbonara

1 Cook the pasta in a large pan of boiling water containing the stock cube.
2 In a separate pan, heat the milk with the garlic. Mix the arrowroot with a little cold milk and whisk into the hot milk.
3 Add the mustard, ham and cheese to the milk. Season with black pepper and add a little more milk if required to adjust the consistency.
4 Drain the pasta and arrange on serving plates. Pour the sauce over and garnish with a little fresh basil.

❄️

SERVES 4
PER SERVING
359 CALORIES
6.9G FAT

PREPARATION TIME 5 MINUTES
COOKING TIME 20 MINUTES

225g tagliatelle
1 vegetable stock cube
600ml semi-skimmed milk
1 garlic clove, crushed
3 teaspoons arrowroot
1 teaspoon Dijon mustard
115g cooked ham
50g Rosemary Conley mature
    cheese, grated
freshly ground black pepper
fresh basil to garnish

TIP *Use a carving fork to loosen the tagliatelle during cooking*

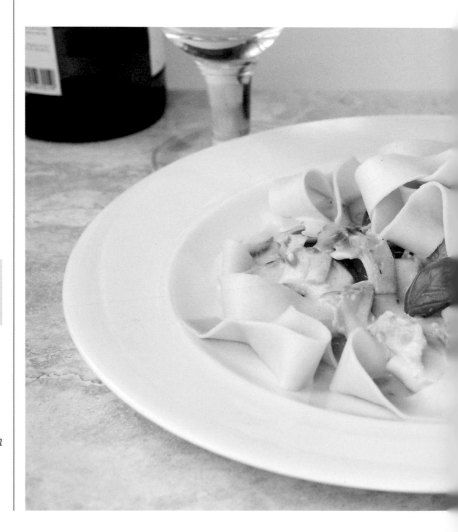

Tagliatelle carbonara

Spicy prawn pasta

1 Cook the pasta shapes in boiling salted water.
2 Meanwhile heat a non-stick frying pan, and dry-fry the red onion for 2–3 minutes until soft. Add the garlic and cook for 2–3 minutes more.
3 Add the tomatoes and chilli, and bring the sauce to a gentle simmer. Add the prawns and season to taste with salt and black pepper. Continue to cook for 3–4 minutes more, making sure the prawns are heated through.
4 Drain the pasta and pour into a serving dish. Spoon the sauce over the pasta and sprinkle with chopped coriander.

SERVES 4
PER SERVING
270 CALORIES
1.6G FAT

PREPARATION TIME 10 MINUTES
COOKING TIME 20 MINUTES

225g (dry weight) pasta shapes
1 red onion, finely chopped
2 garlic cloves, crushed
225g cooked peeled prawns
1 × 400g can chopped
    tomatoes
1 red chilli, deseeded and finely
    chopped
salt and freshly ground black
    pepper
2 tablespoons chopped fresh
    coriander to garnish

TIP *For variations on this pasta dish, try substituting chicken or roasted vegetables for the prawns*

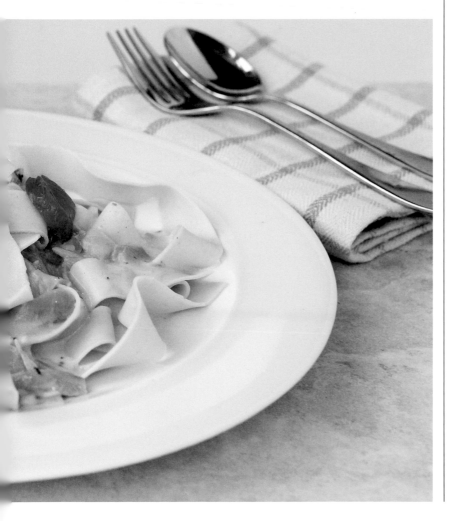

Mushroom and spinach pasta bake

SERVES 4
PER SERVING
369 CALORIES
7.3G FAT

PREPARATION TIME 10 MINUTES
COOKING TIME 20 MINUTES

600ml semi-skimmed milk
4 teaspoons arrowroot
2 teaspoons grainy mustard
1–2 teaspoons vegetable stock
    powder
225g (dry weight) pasta shapes
225g chestnut mushrooms,
    finely chopped
1 garlic clove, crushed
225g fresh spinach, washed
50g low-fat vegetarian
    cheddar-style cheese, grated
freshly ground black pepper

TIP *For a different flavour add a little grated fresh nutmeg to the spinach during cooking*

1 Preheat the oven to 200C, 400F, gas mark 6.
2 Heat the milk in a small saucepan. Mix the arrowroot with a little cold milk then mix into the hot milk, stirring well to prevent any lumps forming. Stir in the mustard and vegetable stock powder, then remove from the heat.
3 Cook the pasta in a pan of boiling water, drain and add to the sauce.
4 Heat a non-stick wok, and dry-fry the mushrooms and garlic until soft. Add the spinach and continue cooking until the spinach is wilted. Add to the sauce along with half the cheese, and season with black pepper.
5 Pour the mixture into an ovenproof dish. Cover with the remaining cheese and bake near the top of the oven for 10 minutes or until golden brown. Serve hot.

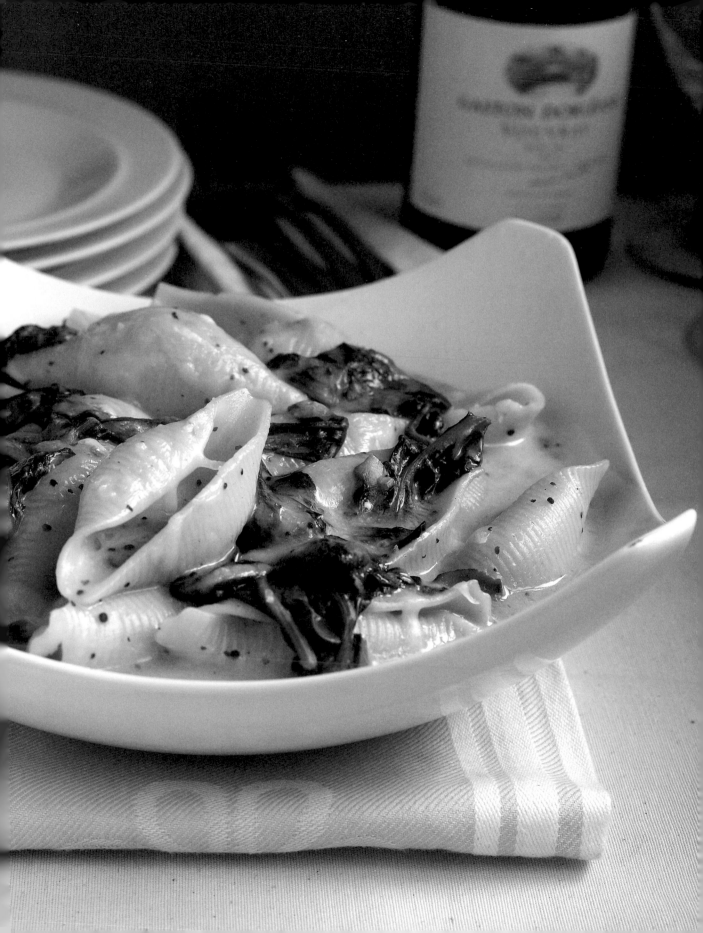

Roweena's healthy pizza

SERVES 4
275 CALORIES
2.4G FAT

PREPARATION TIME 10 MINUTES
COOKING TIME 35 MINUTES

for the dough
225g strong white bread flour
1 teaspoon salt
15g fresh yeast or 2 teaspoons
    dried
150ml warm skimmed milk

for the topping
4 spring onions, finely chopped
1 x 400g can plum tomatoes
12 basil leaves
1 red pepper, deseeded and
    diced
100g mushrooms, sliced
8 cherry tomatoes
50g Rosemary Conley mature
    cheese, grated (available
    from Asda and Morrisons)
1 tablespoon extra light
    mayonnaise

TIP *Drizzling extra light mayonnaise on the cheese helps the cheese to melt into the pizza*

1 Preheat the oven to 200C ,400F, gas mark 6.
2 Place the flour and salt into a large mixing bowl and make a slight well in the centre. Dissolve the yeast in the milk, add to the flour and mix together with the blade of a round-ended knife, adding more liquid if required. Turn out on to a floured surface and knead well to form a soft dough. Cover with a damp cloth for 10 minutes.
3 Place the plum tomatoes (with juice) and 6 basil leaves in a blender (save the remainder for the garnish), and chop roughly.
4 Knead the dough again. Roll it out into a large circle and transfer to a non-stick baking tray or pizza pan. Spoon the tomato mixture over, leaving a border around the edge. Scatter with the onions, pepper, mushrooms and cherry tomatoes, then cover with the grated cheese. Drizzle the mayonnaise over.
5 Place the baking tray or pizza pan on the top shelf of the oven, and bake the pizza for 20 minutes.
6 Shred the remaining basil leaves and scatter over the pizza. Serve hot with a tossed salad.

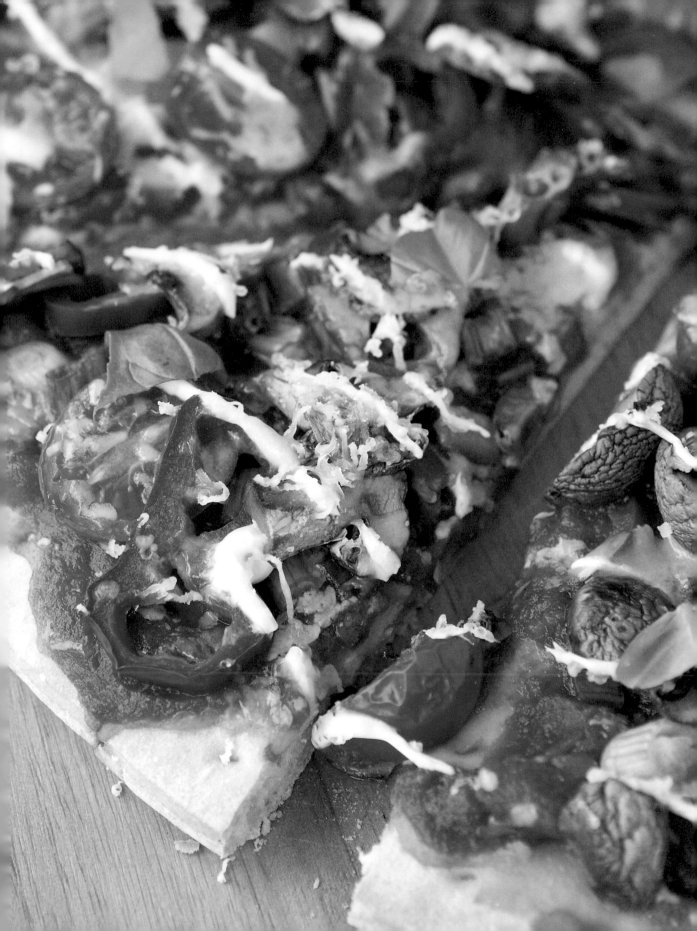

Speedy French bread pizzas

SERVES 2
PER SERVING
296 CALORIES
1.5G FAT

PREPARATION TIME 5 MINUTES
COOKING TIME 20 MINUTES

1 × 150g Bake Off baguette
   (ordinary or gluten free)
4 tablespoons tomato salsa
2 spring onions, finely chopped
1 red pepper, deseeded and
   finely diced
a few fresh basil leaves,
   chopped
50g Rosemary Conley mature
   cheese, grated

1 Preheat the oven to 200C, 400F,
   gas mark 6.
2 Place the baguette on a baking tray
   and bake in the oven for 10
   minutes.
3 When cooked, allow the baguette to
   cool slightly then slice it lengthways
   with a serrated knife. Open out the
   bread and return to the oven for 5
   minutes to lightly toast.
4 Spread the bread with the tomato
   salsa and top with the spring
   onions, red pepper, basil and
   cheese. Return to the oven for 5
   minutes until the cheese has
   melted.

TIP *You can substitute 100g
regular French bread for the
baguette and just put in the
oven or under the grill for 5
minutes to melt the cheese*

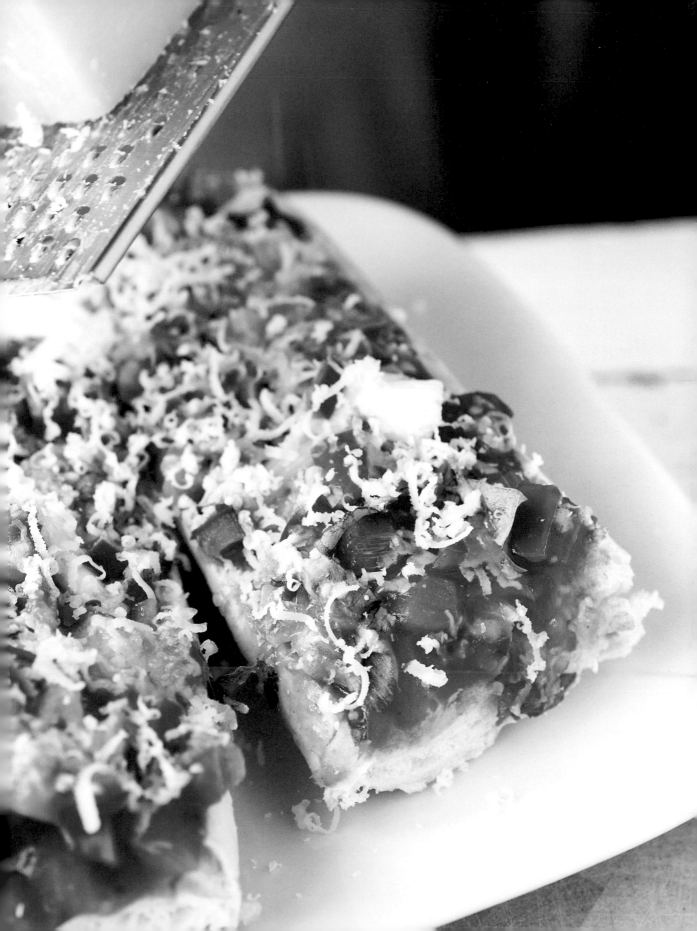

Quorn lasagne verde

SERVES 6
PER SERVING
323 CALORIES
5.7G FAT

PREPARATION TIME 30 MINUTES
COOKING TIME 1 HOUR

2 large red onions, finely diced
2 garlic cloves, crushed
1 × 300g pack frozen Quorn
    mince
1 × 400g can chopped
    tomatoes
1 × 500g pack tomato passata
2 teaspoons chopped fresh
    thyme
1 teaspoon vegetable stock
    powder
250g no pre-cook lasagne verde
    sheets

for the topping
600ml semi-skimmed milk
2 teaspoons English mustard
    powder
1 tablespoon cornflour
30g low-fat vegetarian hard
    cheese, grated
salt and freshly ground black
    pepper

1   Preheat the oven to 180C, 350F, gas mark 4.
2   Heat a large non-stick pan, and dry-fry the onions and garlic until soft. Add the Quorn mince, and cook until brown.
3   Add the remaining ingredients and simmer gently for 20 minutes to allow the flavours to combine while you make the topping.
4   Heat the milk and mustard powder in a saucepan. Dilute the cornflour with a little cold milk and whisk into the milk and mustard. Season with salt and black pepper.
5   Spoon a thin layer of the sauce into an ovenproof dish. Cover with a layer of lasagne sheets (don't overlap them, as they will expand during cooking). Continue layering the Quorn sauce and pasta sheets.
6   Cover the top with the remaining sauce and sprinkle with the grated cheese.
7   Bake in the oven for 35–40 minutes until brown.

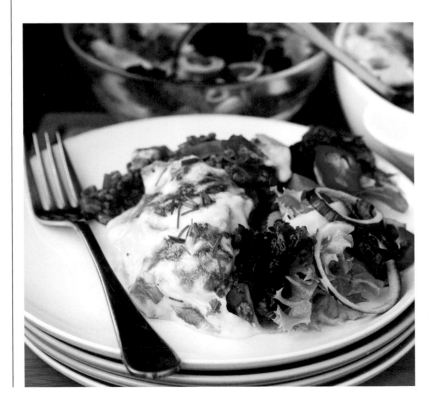

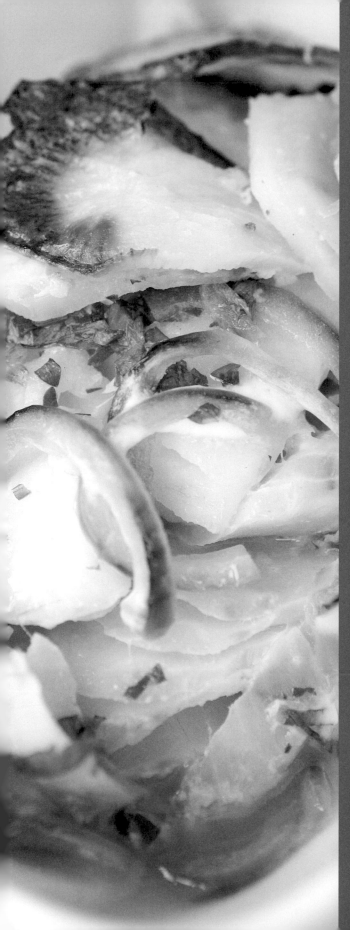

Family favourites

All the family, including the children, will enjoy these delicious dishes and this section offers plenty of variety so you're sure to find something that suits every taste, even for the fussiest of eaters.

Barbecue topped chicken

SERVES 4
PER SERVING
318 CALORIES
8.7G FAT

PREPARATION TIME 10 MINUTES
COOKING TIME 30–35 MINUTES

1 egg, beaten
1 garlic clove, crushed
4 × 125g skinless chicken
    breasts
4 tablespoons fine cornmeal
2 tablespoons barbecue sauce
50g Rosemary Conley mature
    cheese, grated
salt and freshly ground black
    pepper

TIP *For added flavour, add a few chopped fresh chives to the cornmeal*

1 Preheat the oven to 200C, 400F, gas mark 6.
2 Mix together the beaten egg and the garlic in a shallow bowl and season with salt and black pepper. Add the chicken breasts and coat on all sides.
3 Spread out the cornmeal on a plate and roll the chicken in it, pressing the chicken down and coating both sides of the breast.
4 Place the chicken on a non-stick baking tray and bake in the oven for 25–30 minutes, until cooked through.
5 Remove the chicken from the oven, spoon the barbecue sauce over it, then sprinkle with the grated cheese.
6 Return the chicken to the oven for 2–3 minutes to melt the cheese. Serve with salad.

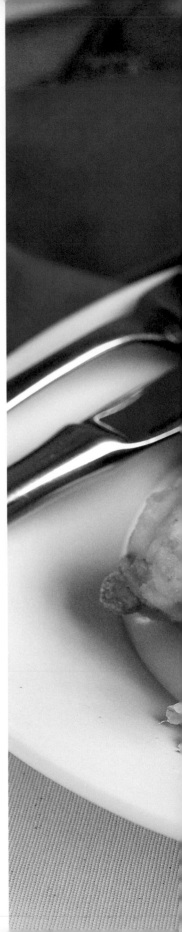

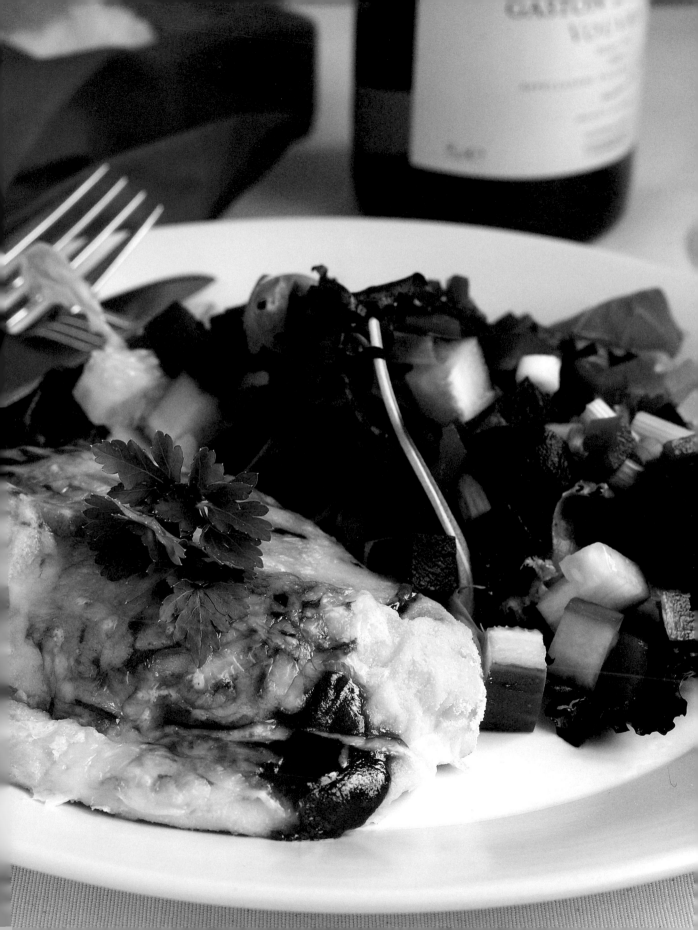

Sage and onion stuffed chicken

SERVES 4
PER SERVING
266 CALORIES
6.1G FAT

PREPARATION TIME 10 MINUTES
COOKING TIME 25 MINUTES

1 medium red onion, finely
    chopped
1 garlic clove, crushed
50g fresh breadcrumbs
1 tablespoon chopped fresh
    sage
150ml hot vegetable stock
salt and freshly ground black
    pepper
4 × 175g skinless chicken
    breasts

TIP *You can substitute 1 teaspoon dried sage for 1 tablespoon chopped fresh sage*

1 Preheat the oven to 200C, 400F, gas mark 6.
2 Heat a non-stick wok or frying pan, and dry-fry the onion and garlic until soft.
3 Add the breadcrumbs and sage, then pour in the hot vegetable stock. Season well, then continue cooking until the mixture firms up. Remove from the heat and allow to cool.
4 Slice each chicken breast across the centre to form a pocket in each one, and place on a non-stick baking tray. Fill the chicken breasts with some of the stuffing, and spread the remainder over the top. Bake in the oven for 20–25 minutes until cooked through. Serve with fresh vegetables of your choice.

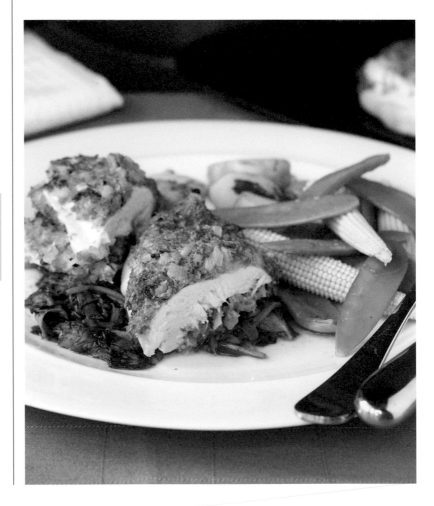

Braised turkey and pork rolls

1. Preheat the oven to 180C, 350F, gas mark 4.
2. In a small bowl, mix the minced pork with 1 crushed garlic clove and half the mixed herbs. Season with black pepper.
3. Place the turkey steaks on a chopping board. Spoon a quarter of the pork mixture on to each steak, then and roll up the steaks, encasing the pork mixture.
4. Heat a heavy-based, non-stick pan, and dry-fry the turkey rolls until brown all over. Transfer to an ovenproof dish.
5. Stir the onions and remaining garlic into the hot pan, and cook until soft. Add the stock, white wine and tomato passata, then pour the sauce over the turkey.
6. Cover, and braise in the oven for 30 minutes or until the meat is tender. Sprinkle with the parsley and serve with 100g dry-roasted sweet potatoes per person, Courgette and Pepper Rosti (see recipe page 247) and green vegetables.

SERVES 4
PER SERVING
203 CALORIES
2.2G FAT

PREPARATION TIME 15 MINUTES
COOKING TIME 40 MINUTES

100g lean minced pork
2 garlic cloves, crushed
2 tablespoons chopped fresh mixed herbs (e.g. rosemary, thyme, oregano)
4 × 100g thin-cut turkey steaks
2 medium red onions, finely chopped
300ml chicken stock
120ml white wine
300g tomato passata
freshly ground black pepper
2 tablespoons chopped fresh parsley to garnish

TIP *To get the turkey steaks thin, place them between 2 sheets of clingfilm and beat with a rolling pin*

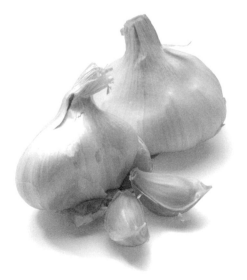

Lamb and pepper hotpot

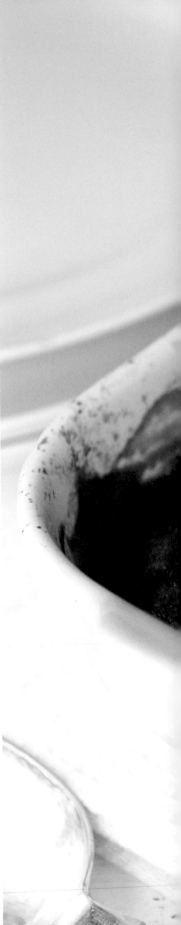

❄️

SERVES 4
PER SERVING
372 CALORIES
17G FAT

PREPARATION TIME 10 MINUTES
COOKING TIME 45 MINUTES

450g lean diced lamb
1 medium red onion, finely
    chopped
2 garlic cloves, crushed
1 red pepper, deseeded and
    diced
500g tomato passata
2 teaspoons vegetable stock
    powder, dissolved in 300ml
    water
1 tablespoon chopped fresh
    mixed herbs
2 tablespoons chopped fresh
    mint
2 sweet potatoes, peeled and
    sliced
1 vegetable stock cube
freshly ground black pepper

TIP *This recipe is ideal for cooking in a slow cooker*

1 Preheat the oven to 200C, 400F, gas mark 6.
2 Heat a heavy-based, non-stick pan. Season the lamb with black pepper, add to the hot pan and seal the meat on all sides.
3 Add the onion, garlic and red pepper, and cook quickly over a high heat until soft.
4 Add the tomato passata, made-up stock and the herbs, stirring well. Cover and simmer for 30 minutes to allow the lamb to cook through.
5 Meanwhile, cook the sweet potato slices in a pan of water with the vegetable stock cube.
6 When the meat is tender, stir in the chopped mint and pour into an ovenproof dish. Drain the potatoes and arrange on top of the meat.
7 Bake in the oven for 15–20 minutes until golden.

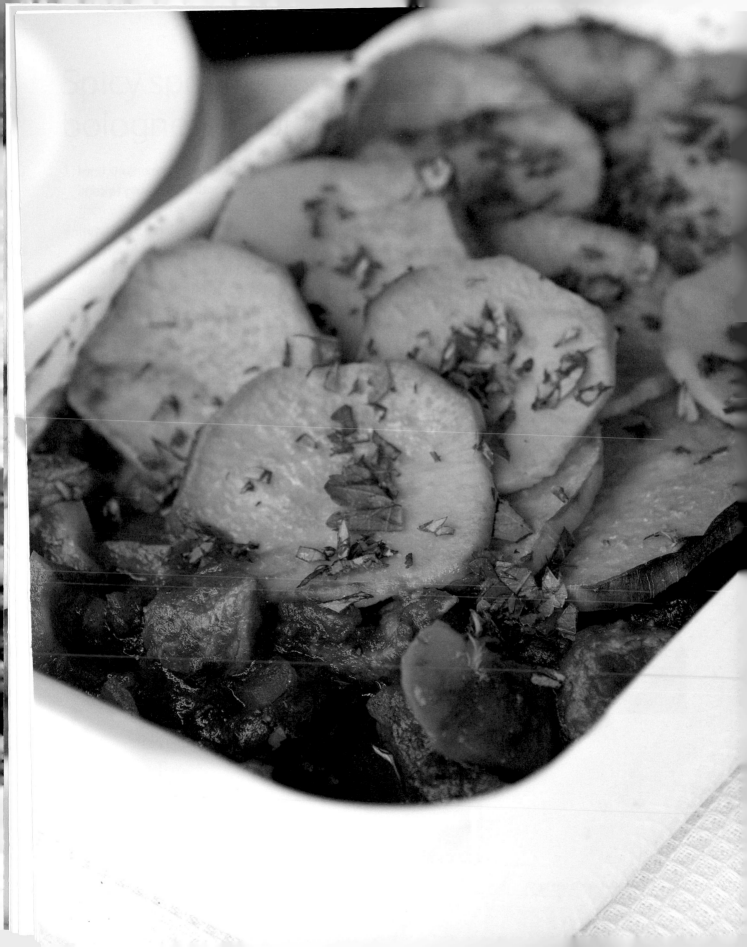

Quorn sausage casserole

SERVES 2
PER SERVING
221 CALORIES
6.9G FAT

PREPARATION TIME 10 MINUTES
COOKING TIME 10 MINUTES

250g Quorn Cumberland
 sausages
1 red onion, sliced
1 tablespoon chopped fresh
 thyme
1 teaspoon wholegrain mustard
2 tablespoons red wine
1 × 400g can chopped
 tomatoes
freshly ground black pepper

TIP *As an alternative you can substitute Quorn fillets or meatballs for the sausages*

1 Heat a non-stick frying pan, and dry-fry the sausages until lightly browned. Add the sliced onion and continue cooking until soft.
2 Add the remaining ingredients and bring to a gentle simmer. Cover and simmer for 10 minutes until the sausages are cooked through.
3 Just before serving, season with black pepper and serve with vegetables of your choice.

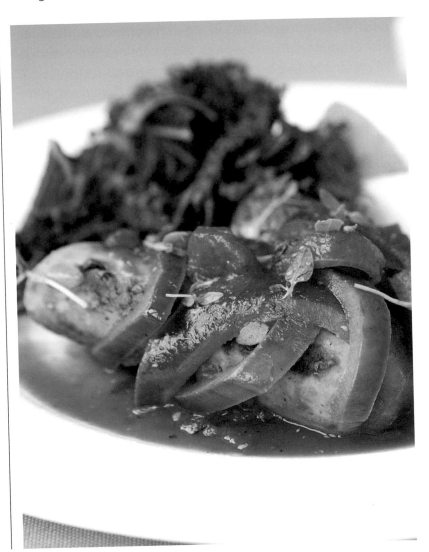

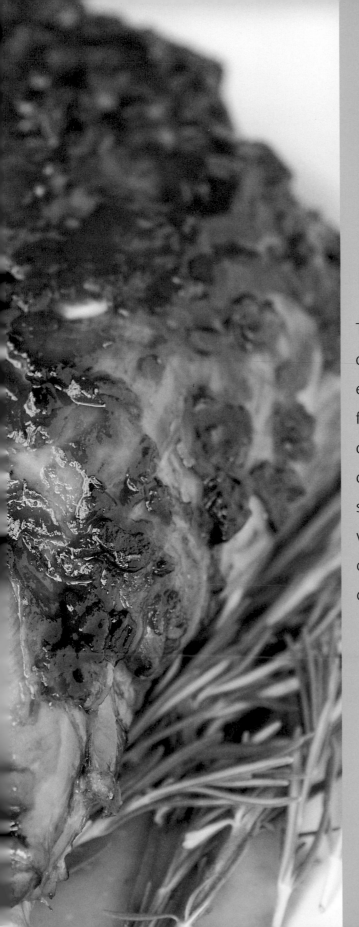

Really easy roasts

There's nothing quite like getting family and friends together round the table and enjoying a traditional roast. These five flavoursome dishes show how you can add interest in the form of herbs, coatings and marinades and they're all really simple to prepare. Just add your choice of vegetable accompaniments, and check out the recipe for low-fat Roast Parsnips and Sweet Potatoes on page 225.

Herb-crusted lamb fillet

SERVES 4
PER SERVING
234 CALORIES
16.4G FAT

PREPARATION TIME 10 MINUTES
COOKING TIME 20 MINUTES

1 × 450g piece lean lamb fillet
1 tablespoon mint sauce
2 tablespoons chopped fresh
    herbs (e.g. thyme, parsley,
    basil)
salt and freshly ground black
    pepper

TIP *For a quick gravy, while the meat is resting add 600ml water to the cooking dish, bring to the boil and thicken with a few gravy granules or gravy powder*

1 Preheat the oven to 200C, 400F, gas mark 6.
2 Remove any remaining visible fat from the lamb with a sharp knife.
3 Scatter the herbs in the base of an ovenproof dish and season well with salt and black pepper.
4 Using a knife, spread the mint sauce over the lamb and then roll the lamb in the herbs. Pat the herbs on to the lamb, making sure they stick to the mint sauce.
5 Roast near the top of the oven for 15–20 minutes, until cooked to your liking, then remove from the oven and allow it to rest for 5 minutes before carving. Serve with couscous and steamed green vegetables.

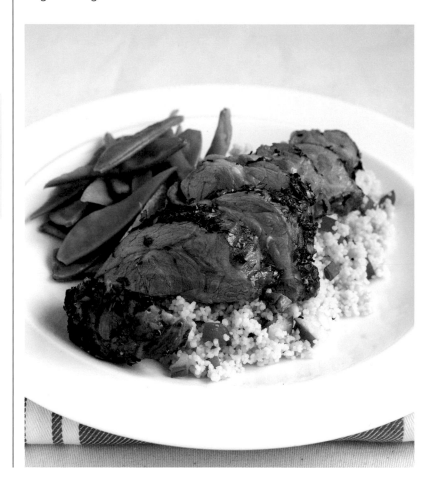

Honey and lemon roast chicken

1 Preheat the oven to 200C, 400F, gas mark 6
2 Cut the lemon in half. Season the chicken breasts on both sides with salt and black pepper and place in a non-stick roasting tin.
3 Squeeze the lemon juice over the chicken and place the lemon flesh under each chicken breast. Drizzle with the honey and roast in the oven for 25–30 minutes until cooked. Serve with dry-roasted vegetables.

SERVES 2
PER SERVING
249 KCAL
3.3G FAT

PREPARATION TIME 10 MINUTES
COOKING TIME 25–30 MINUTES

2 × 150g chicken breasts
juice of 1 lemon
2 teaspoons runny honey
salt and freshly ground black
    pepper

TIP *You can also use chicken quarters. Remember to trim away as much skin as possible*

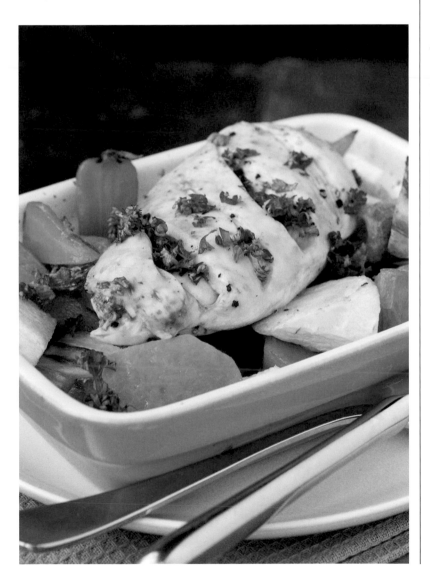

Cider roast chicken

❄️

SERVES 4
PER SERVING
165 CALORIES
1.9G FAT

PREPARATION TIME 10 MINUTES
COOKING TIME 30 MINUTES

8 chicken legs, skin removed
4 long shallots, peeled and
    sliced in half
2 garlic cloves, sliced
3 celery sticks, chopped
1 tablespoon fresh thyme or
    sage leaves
300ml cider
2 tablespoons chopped fresh
    parsley
1 teaspoon gravy powder
salt and freshly ground black
    pepper

TIP *For a fuller flavour,
marinate the ingredients
overnight in the refrigerator
before roasting*

1 Preheat the oven to 200C, 400F, gas
   mark 6.
2 Place the chicken, shallots, garlic and
   celery in a non-stick roasting tin. Add
   the thyme or sage leaves and drizzle
   the cider over the chicken pieces.
   Season with salt and black pepper.
3 Cover the chicken with foil and roast
   in the centre of the oven for 30
   minutes. Five minutes before the
   end of cooking, remove the foil to
   brown the chicken. Transfer the
   chicken to a serving dish, and
   thicken the sauce in the roasting tin
   with a little gravy powder.
4 Pour the sauce over the chicken and
   sprinkle with chopped fresh parsley.

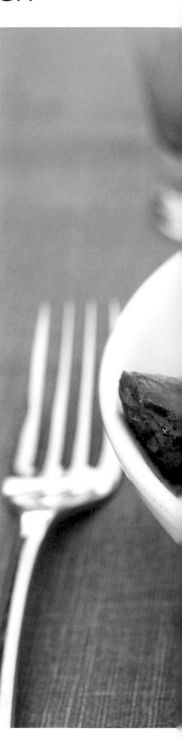

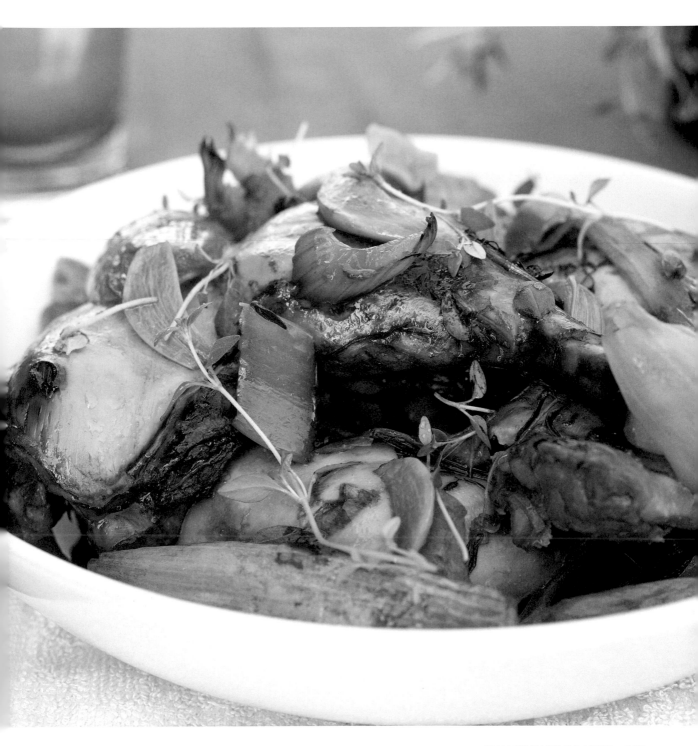

REALLY EASY ROASTS 157

Roast lamb with honey and rosemary glaze

SERVES 8
PER SERVING
254 CALORIES
16G FAT

PREPARATION TIME 10 MINUTES
COOKING TIME 1–1½ HOURS

2 tablespoons runny honey
2 garlic cloves, crushed
3–4 sprigs fresh rosemary, chopped
zest and juice of 1 lemon
1 tablespoons tomato purée
1 × 1kg leg of lamb, all visible fat removed
600ml water
2 teaspoons gravy powder
2 teaspoons finely chopped fresh mint
freshly ground black pepper

TIP *Leave the meat to rest for 10 minutes to allow it to relax before carving*

1 Preheat the oven to 180C, 350F, gas mark 4. Put a rack in a non-stick roasting tin for the lamb to sit on.
2 In a small bowl, mix together the honey, garlic, rosemary, lemon zest and juice and tomato purée.
3 Make small incisions all over the lamb, using a small knife, then place the lamb on the rack inside the roasting tin. Using a brush, paste the marinade over the lamb, pushing it into the holes, then season with black pepper. Pour the water into the base of the roasting tin to prevent the juices from burning. Cover the lamb with foil and place in the oven for 1–1½ hours until tender.
4 When the lamb is cooked, strain the juices into a gravy separator. Pour out the fat from the roasting tin and top up the tin with more water. Thicken with a little gravy powder and stir in the chopped mint.

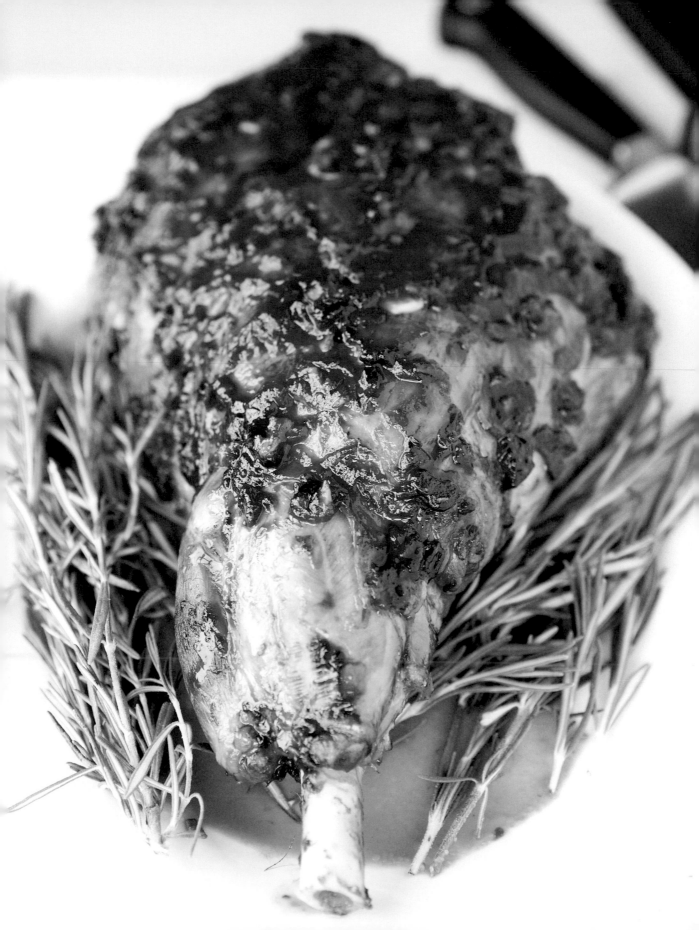

Stuffed pork fillet

SERVES 4
PER SERVING
270 KCAL
10.5G FAT

PREPARATION TIME 10 MINUTES
COOKING TIME 25–30 MINUTES

1 × 450g piece lean pork fillet
120g Quark soft cheese
1 tablespoon chopped fresh
   chives
1 garlic clove, crushed
200g pancetta
salt and freshly ground black
   pepper

TIP *Fresh basil is a good
substitute for chives*

1 Preheat the oven to 200C, 400F, gas mark 6.
2 Remove any remaining visible fat from the pork. Place the pork on a chopping board. Using a sharp knife, cut the fillet down the centre but not all the way through. Open up the pork to form a flat piece of meat.
3 Mix together the Quark, chives and garlic and season with salt and black pepper. Spread the Quark mixture over the pork and roll up the pork.
4 Wrap the pancetta around the rolled-up pork and place in a non-stick roasting tray. Roast in the oven for 20–25 minutes until fully cooked.
5 Remove from the oven and allow it to rest for 5 minutes before carving. Serve with a selection of vegetables.

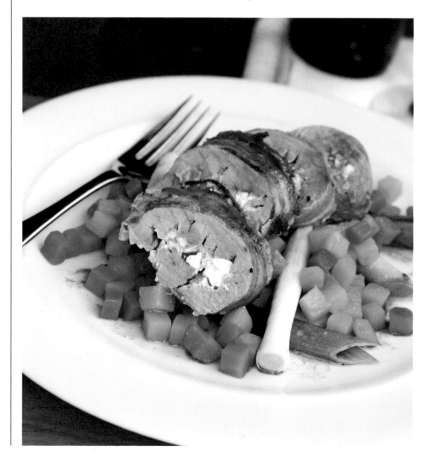

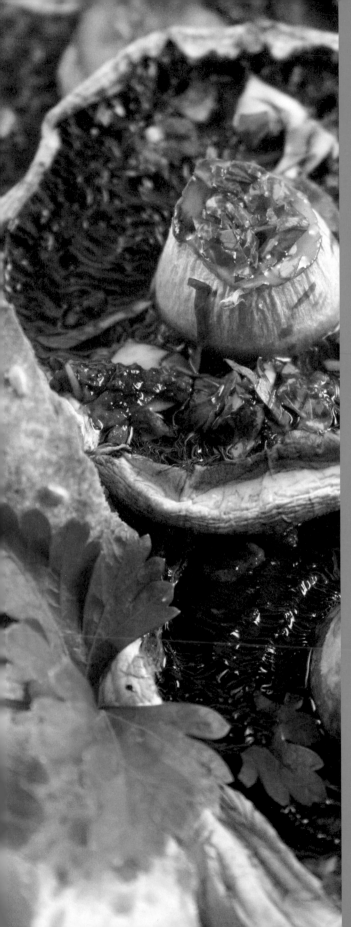

Meals for one

If you're a solo slimmer it can be hard to find recipes that cater for just one person, so here are some suggestions for single-serving meals as well as ideas for tasty toast toppers and jacket potato fillings. Many of the other recipes in this book can be made for two or four people and the other portions frozen for another time, so they're also suitable for one. Just look out for the ❄ symbol, which indicates that they can be frozen.

Quorn stuffed pepper

SERVES 1
PER SERVING
234 CALORIES
6.8G FAT

PREPARATION TIME 20 MINUTES
COOKING TIME 10–15 MINUTES

1 red pepper
75g Quorn mince
1 red onion, finely diced
1 garlic clove, crushed
2 teaspoons chopped fresh
   thyme
½ teaspoon paprika
1 × 200g can tomatoes
½ teaspoon vegetable stock
   powder or to taste
a few fresh basil leaves
1 tablespoon grated low-fat
   vegetarian cheese
freshly ground black pepper

TIP *Serve with salad or
vegetables of your choice for
lunch. If you want, substitute
40g extra lean minced beef for
the Quorn mince*

1 Preheat the oven to 200C, 400F, gas mark 6.
2 Cut the pepper in half, scoop out the seeds and discard.
2 Heat a non-stick pan, and dry-fry the mince, onion and garlic for
   4–5 minutes. Stir in the thyme and paprika and continue
   cooking for 2 minutes.
3 Stir in the tomatoes, stock powder and basil leaves and simmer
   for 5 minutes. Spoon the mixture into the pepper shells.
4 Bake near the top of the oven for 10–15 minutes until the
   peppers are soft. Five minutes before the end of cooking, top
   with the grated cheese and return to the oven.

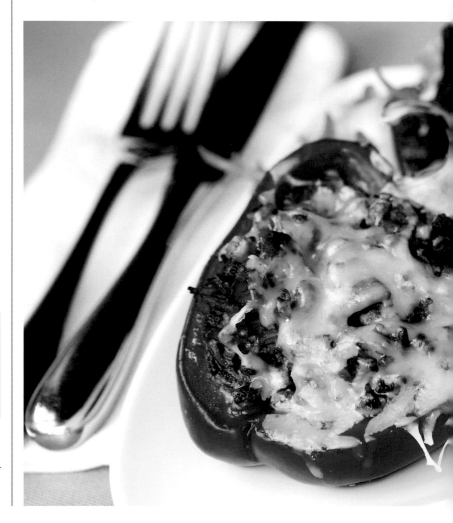

Quorn stuffed pepper

Turkey stir-fry with noodles

1. Cook the noodles in a pan of boiling water with the vegetable stock cube.
2. While the noodles are cooking, heat a non-stick frying pan and lightly spray with oil spray. Add the turkey strips, chilli, ginger and pepper and cook for 3–4 minutes.
3. Add the vegetable stir-fry mix and pak choi and cook for 3 minutes. Season with the lime juice and soy sauce.
4. Drain the noodles and transfer to a serving plate. Spoon the turkey mixture over.

SERVES 1
PER SERVING
417 CALORIES
5.7G FAT

PREPARATION TIME 10 MINUTES
COOKING TIME 15–20 MINUTES

40g (dry weight) Chinese egg noodles
1 vegetable stock cube
low-calorie oil spray
150g skinless turkey breast, cut into strips
1 red chilli, deseeded and finely chopped
1 × 2cm piece fresh ginger, grated
1 yellow pepper, cut into strips
75g vegetable stir-fry mix
50g pak choi
juice of ½ lime
2 teaspoons soy sauce

TIP *You can use any mixture of vegetables or buy a pack of ready-chopped ones*

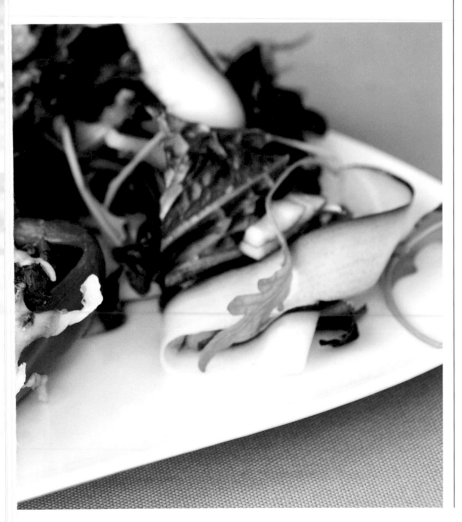

Fruity coleslaw ☑

Mix ½ grated eating apple, 1 small grated carrot, and 1 small grated courgette with 1 tablespoon of extra light mayonnaise.

PER SERVING (INCLUDING POTATO)
235 CALORIES
2G FAT

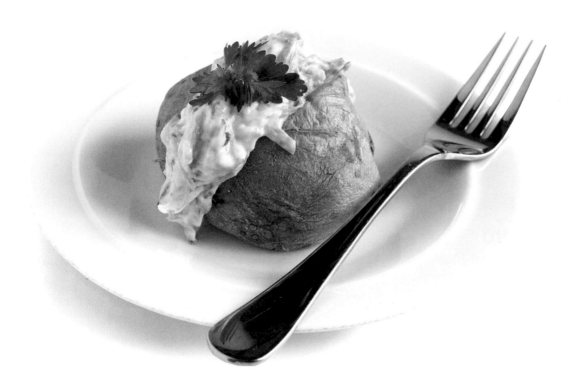

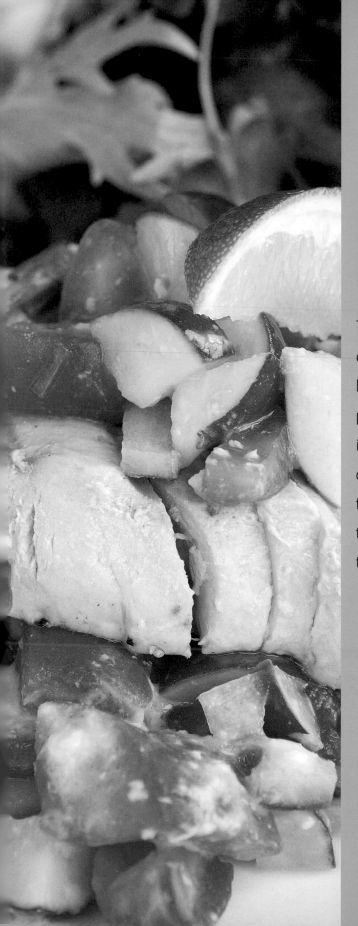

20-minute meals

These super-quick meals are ideal for days when you're pushed for time but have nothing suitable in the freezer. Or perhaps you need to rustle up an impromptu supper for friends. They can all can be prepared and cooked from fresh in 20 minutes or less, from kitchen to table. All calorie and fat counts include the suggested accompaniments.

Pan-fried beef with brandy

SERVES 4
PER SERVING
416 CALORIES
8.2G FAT

PREPARATION TIME 10 MINUTES
COOKING TIME 20 MINUTES

1 × 100g piece granary French
    stick
1 garlic clove, crushed
4 × 150g beef rump steaks,
    thinly sliced
2 salad onions, finely chopped
2 teaspoons ground coriander
200g pack chestnut
    mushrooms, sliced
150ml beef stock
2 tablespoons brandy
300ml 2% fat Greek yogurt
2 teaspoons Dijon mustard
1 tablespoon chopped fresh
    chives
salt and freshly ground black
    pepper

for serving
400g new potatoes, scrubbed
green vegetables of your choice

TIP *Toss the beef lightly in the pan as it will continue to cook while you prepare the sauce*

Pan-fried beef with brandy

1 Put the potatoes in a pan of boiling water to cook while you prepare the beef. Put the green vegetables in a colander over the pan of boiling water (or use a steamer).
2 Cut the bread into 4 slices. Spread with a little of the crushed garlic (save the remainder) and lightly toast to form croûtes.
3 Heat a large, non-stick frying pan, and quickly toss the rump steaks in the pan to seal them, seasoning with salt and black pepper. Remove from the pan and set aside.
4 Add the onions, coriander, mushrooms and remaining garlic to the pan. Pour in the beef stock and brandy, taking care not to let the brandy flame in the pan. If it does, just leave it to burn off the alcohol. Keep cooking as the stock reduces.
5 Return the steaks to the pan, then stir in the yogurt, mustard and chives.
6 Drain the potatoes, then serve each steak on a croûte alongside the potatoes and the steamed greens.

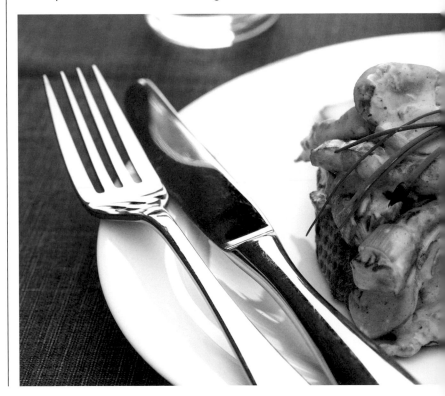

Pork with balsamic peppers and noodles

1 Heat a non-stick wok. Cut the pork steaks into strips.
2 Add the onion and garlic to the hot wok and dry-fry until soft. Add the pork and peppers, tossing well. When the meat is sealed, add the balsamic vinegar and honey.
3 Add the pak choi or spinach and season with a little salt and plenty of black pepper.
4 Meanwhile, cook the noodles in boiling water or as directed on the packet, then drain.
5 Serve the pork on a bed of noodles.

SERVES 4
PER SERVING
389 CALORIES
5.6G FAT

PREPARATION TIME 10 MINUTES
COOKING TIME 20 MINUTES

4 × 120g lean pork steaks, all
    visible fat removed
1 medium red onion, finely
    chopped
1 garlic clove, crushed
1 red and 1 yellow pepper,
    deseeded and diced
1 tablespoon good balsamic
    vinegar
1 tablespoon runny honey
200g pak choi or spinach
salt and freshly ground black
    pepper
200g (dry weight) noodles

TIP *Cut the pork into similar-sized strips to ensure they cook evenly*

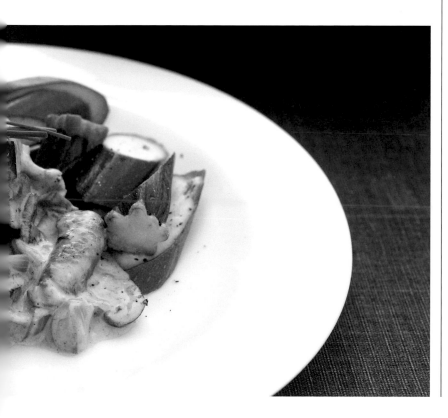

Pork and pineapple burgers

SERVES 4
PER SERVING
325 CALORIES
6.9G FAT

PREPARATION TIME 10 MINUTES
COOKING TIME 20 MINUTES

450g lean minced pork
2 teaspoons vegetable stock
    powder
1 × 137g can chopped
    pineapple, drained
1 tablespoon chilli sauce
4 spring onions, finely chopped
freshly ground black pepper

for serving
4 wholegrain rolls
salad leaves
4 tablespoons tomato salsa

TIP *You can substitute minced chicken or turkey for the pork*

1 Preheat a conventional or health grill.
2 Place all the ingredients in a mixing bowl and season with black pepper. Shape the mixture into 4 burgers.
3 Cook the burgers under the hot grill or in a health grill for 10–15 minutes, turning regularly. Test to see if they are cooked through to the centre by inserting a knife.
4 Serve each burger in a wholegrain roll with salad leaves and tomato salsa.

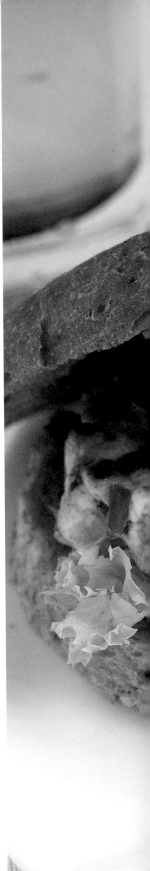

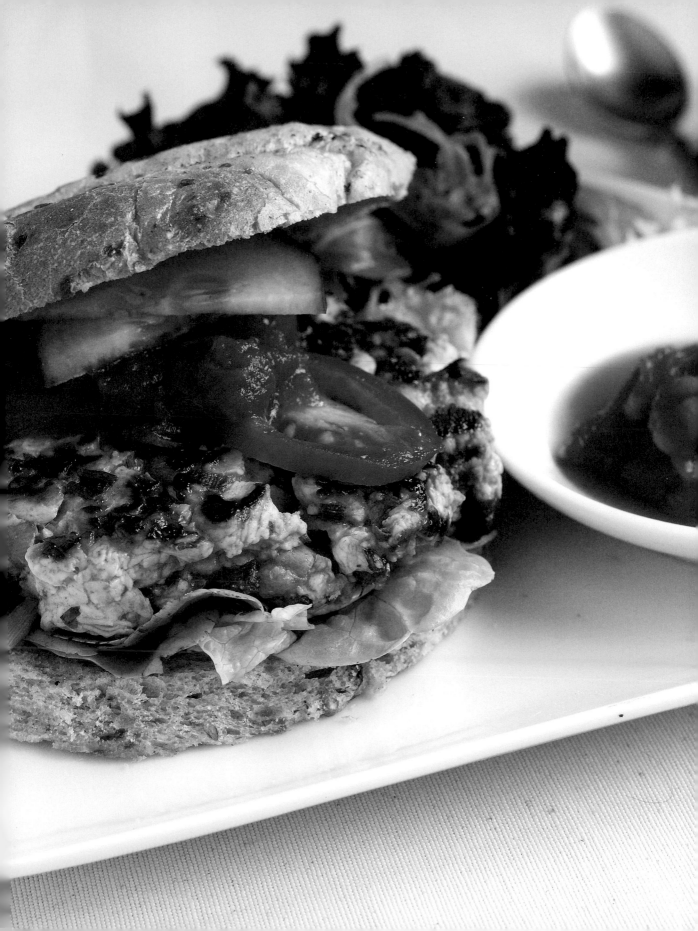

Lamb with red wine

SERVES 4
PER SERVING
168 CALORIES
5.1G FAT

PREPARATION TIME 10 MINUTES
COOKING TIME 20 MINUTES

1 medium onion, finely
    chopped
2 garlic cloves, crushed
225g lean lamb steak, diced
1–2 teaspoons vegetable stock
    powder
1 tablespoon plain flour
150ml red wine
1 × 400g can chopped
    tomatoes
110g button mushrooms
1 tablespoon chopped fresh
    thyme
salt and freshly ground black
    pepper
1 tablespoon chopped fresh
    parsley to garnish

TIP *Choose very lean cuts of
lamb. Leg steaks are leaner
than shoulder steaks*

1 Heat a non-stick frying pan, and dry-
   fry the chopped onion and garlic
   until soft.
2 Add the diced lamb to the pan to
   lightly colour it and season with salt
   and black pepper. Add the stock
   powder, sprinkle the flour over and
   continue cooking for 1 minute.
3 Gradually stir in the wine and the
   remaining ingredients. Reduce the
   heat and simmer gently for 20
   minutes until the lamb is tender.
4 Just before serving sprinkle with the
   chopped parsley. Serve with a
   selection of fresh vegetables.

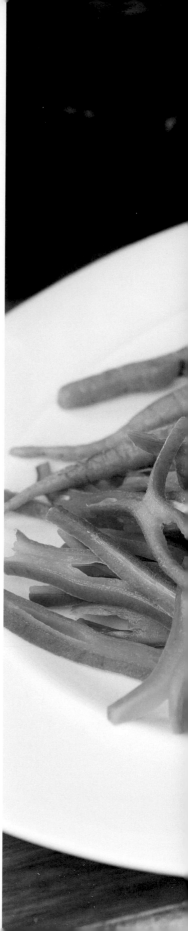

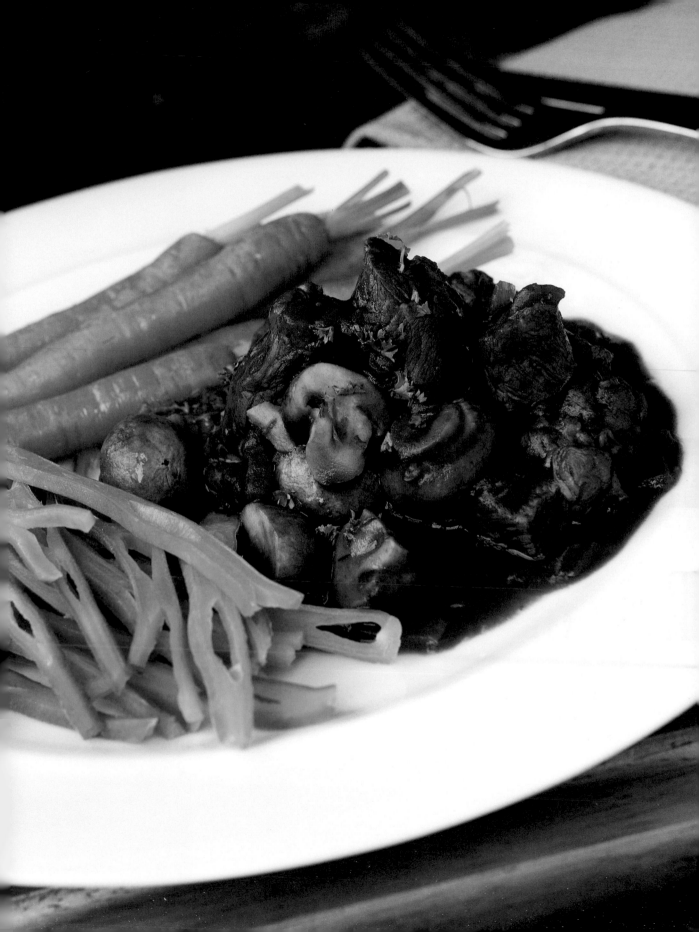

Pan-fried liver with leek mash

SERVES 2
PER SERVING
228 CALORIES
7.7G FAT

PREPARATION TIME 10 MINUTES
COOKING TIME 20 MINUTES

200g potatoes
200g green vegetables of your
   choice
1 leek sliced
400g sliced lamb's liver
1 red onion, sliced
1 tablespoon chopped fresh
   thyme
2 tablespoons red wine
150ml water
1–2 teaspoons gravy powder
1 teaspoon wholegrain mustard
freshly ground black pepper

TIP *Do not overcook the liver
or it will become tough*

1 Peel the potatoes and boil in a pan
   of water, adding the sliced leek 5
   minutes before the end of cooking.
   Put the green vegetables in a
   steamer or in a metal colander over
   a pan of boiling water to steam
   while you prepare the pork.
2 Heat a non-stick frying pan, and dry-
   fry the liver until lightly browned.
   Season with black pepper, then
   remove from the pan and keep
   warm.
3 Add the onion to the pan and cook
   until soft. Add the thyme and red
   wine, and stir to deglaze the pan.
   Pour in the water and bring to a
   simmer.
4 Mix the gravy powder with a little
   cold water and whisk into the sauce.
5 Drain the potatoes and leeks, then
   add the mustard and salt and black
   pepper to taste and mash well.
6 Spoon the mash on to serving
   plates. Top with the liver, drizzle the
   gravy over and serve with the
   steamed vegetables.

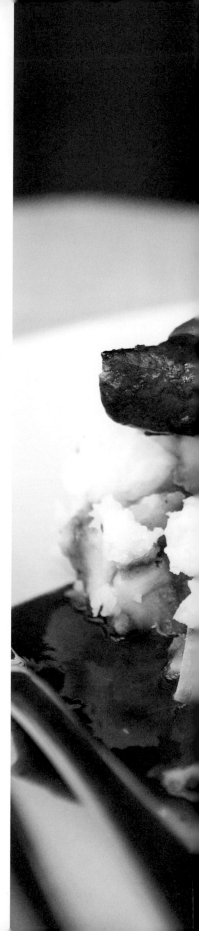

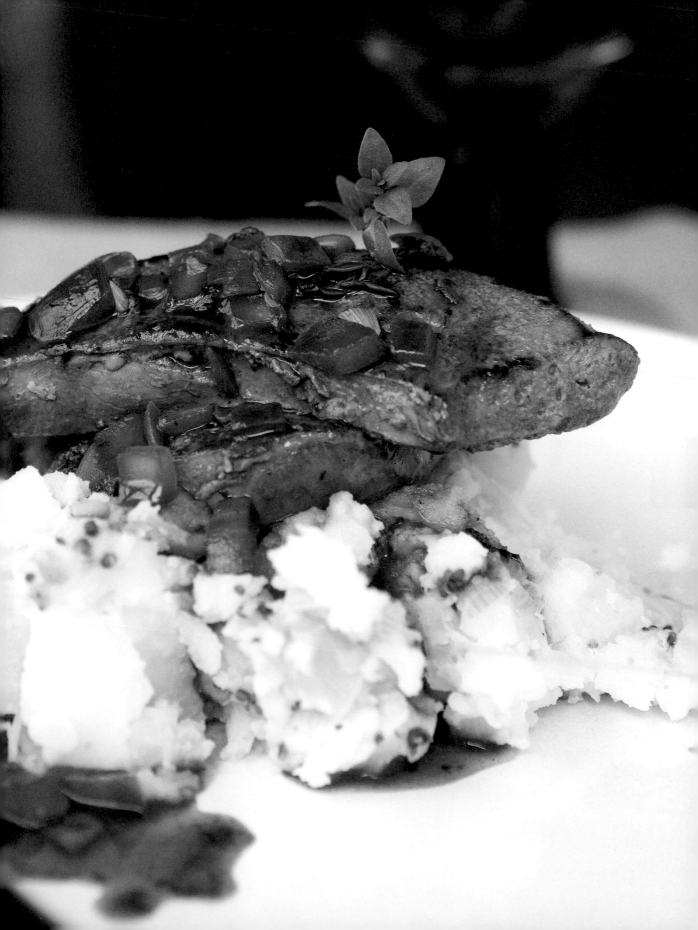

Peppered salmon with noodles

SERVES 4
PER SERVING
400 CALORIES
17.5G FAT

PREPARATION TIME 5 MINUTES
COOKING TIME 15–20 MINUTES

low-calorie oil spray
80g noodles
4 × 150g salmon fillets
4 teaspoons grainy mustard
salt and freshly ground black
    pepper
green salad leaves to serve

for garnishing
2 tablespoons low-fat natural
    yogurt
sprig of fresh mint

TIP *You can wrap these salmon fillets in foil, then cook in a moderate oven and allow to cool for a picnic dish or packed lunch*

1 Preheat a non-stick frying pan and lightly spray with oil spray. Put the noodles in a pan of boiling water to cook while you prepare the salmon.
2 Season the salmon fillets with salt and plenty black pepper, then using a knife, spread the mustard over the top of each fillet.
3 Cook the salmon fillets skin-side down in the frying pan for 7–8 minutes over a moderate heat. Flip the salmon over and continue cooking for 7 minutes. Reduce the heat and cover with a lid to allow the fish to steam and finish cooking.
4 Drain the noodles and arrange in a serving dish. Top with the salmon fillets. Garnish with the yogurt and some fresh mint, and serve with green salad leaves.

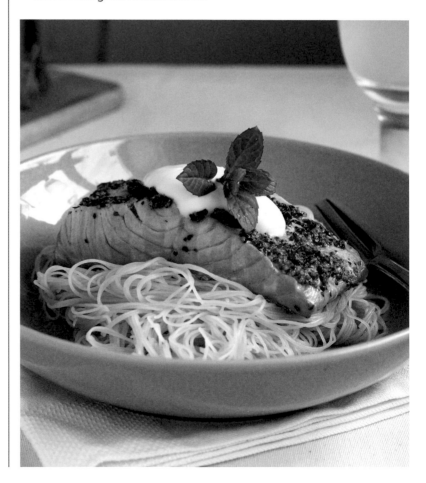

Prawn cocktail pasta

1 Cook the pasta in a pan of boiling water with the vegetable stock cube.
2 Meanwhile, heat the milk in a saucepan. Slake the arrowroot with a little cold water and whisk into the hot milk. Add the remaining ingredients and season with a little black pepper.
3 Drain the pasta well, toss in the sauce and serve with salad.

SERVES 4
PER SERVING
362 CALORIES
3.7G FAT

PREPARATION TIME 10 MINUTES
COOKING TIME 20 MINUTES

225g (dry weight) pasta shapes
1 vegetable stock cube
660ml skimmed milk
2 teaspoons arrowroot
1 teaspoon finely chopped
     lemongrass
1 teaspoon vegetable stock
     powder
1 tablespoon tomato purée
175g cooked peeled prawns
freshly ground black pepper
a few fresh chives to garnish
mixed salad of your choice to
     serve

TIP *Add the prawns at the last minute so you don't overcook them*

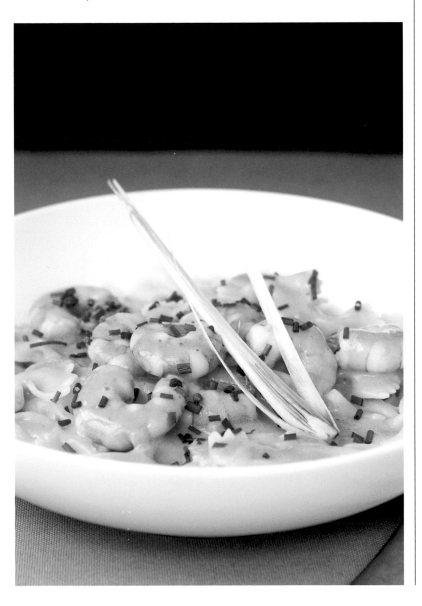

Fresh tuna with tomato and radish salsa

SERVES 4
PER SERVING
381 CALORIES
6.2G FAT

PREPARATION TIME 10 MINUTES
COOKING TIME 20 MINUTES

low-calorie oil spray
4 × 120g fresh tuna steaks
salt and freshly ground black
     pepper

for the salsa
1 small red onion, finely diced
2 beef tomatoes, skinned,
     deseeded and diced
small bunch of radishes,
     chopped
1 tablespoon finely chopped
     chives
2 teaspoons horseradish sauce

for serving
220g (dry weight) basmati rice
salad leaves

TIP *As the tuna steaks cook
you should see them change
colour as the heat rises
through the fish*

1 Preheat a non-stick frying pan and lightly spray with oil spray.
   Put the rice in a pan of boiling water to cook while you prepare
   the tuna.
2 Season the tuna steaks with salt and black pepper. Add to the
   hot frying pan and cook for 2–3 minutes on each side. Remove
   from the heat and keep warm.
3 To make the salsa, add the onion to the pan and cook until soft.
   Add the tomatoes and radishes, then cook for a further 2
   minutes. Remove from the heat and stir in the chives and
   horseradish sauce.
4 Drain the rice, and serve the tuna on a bed of rice with the salsa
   on top and salad leaves alongside.

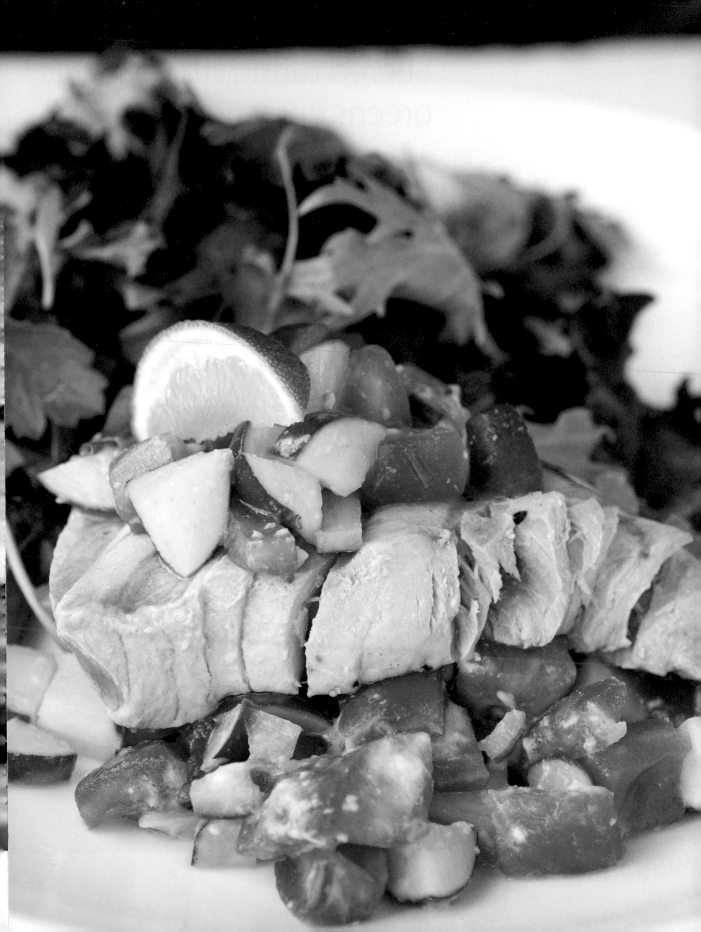

Pasta piperade

SERVES 4
PER SERVING
400 CALORIES
2.1G FAT

PREPARATION TIME 5 MINUTES
COOKING TIME 20 MINUTES

300g (dry weight) pasta shells
1 vegetable stock cube
1 red onion, finely chopped
1 garlic clove, crushed
1 red and 1 yellow pepper,
    deseeded and diced
500g tomato passata
1 small red chilli, sliced
a few fresh basil leaves,
    shredded
freshly ground black pepper to
    taste
green salad to serve

TIP *You can make this pepper sauce in large batches and freeze it*

1 Cook the pasta in a large pan of boiling water with the vegetable stock cube.
2 Heat a non-stick frying pan, and dry-fry the onion and garlic until soft. Add the peppers and cook for 1–2 minutes. Add the tomato passata and chilli and heat through.
3 Drain the pasta and mix with the sauce. Stir in the basil leaves and serve with a green salad.

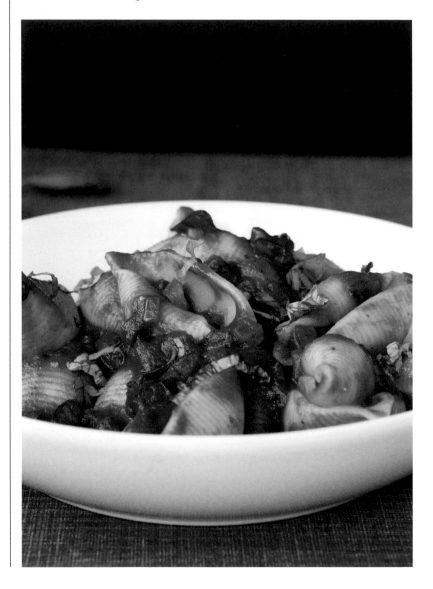

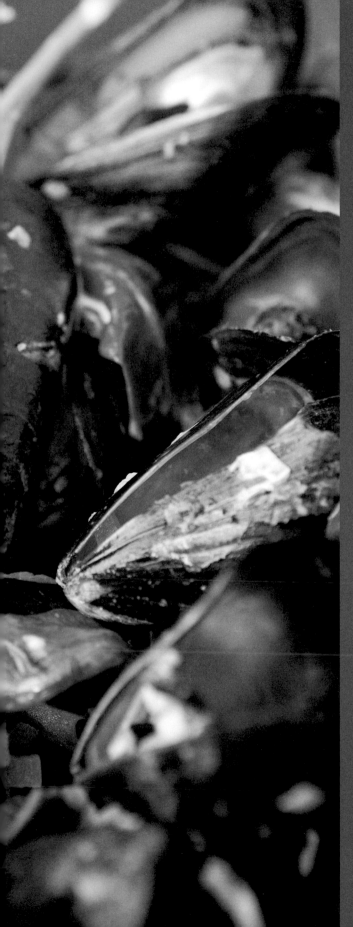

Wine and dine

When you're planning a dinner party or a stylish supper with friends and you want to go that extra mile, you'll find these main course recipes should do the trick. For each recipe, I've given some general suggestions for wine choices to accompany them. Remember, even if you still have some excess pounds to shed, you can enjoy a small glass each day once you've completed the Fat Attack Fortnight Diet.

Some of the party food ideas in chapter 17 double as good, low-calorie starters or take a look at the soups in chapter 5. For vegetable side dishes check out chapter 18 or, for salads, turn to chapter 7. And you're sure to find a pudding to suit in chapter 20.

Cajun duck with mango

SERVES 4
PER SERVING
209 CALORIES
8G FAT

PREPARATION TIME 10 MINUTES
COOKING TIME 20 MINUTES

4 × 120g duck breasts
½ teaspoon cayenne pepper
2 teaspoons ground cumin
2 teaspoons paprika
1 tablespoon chopped fresh
   parsley
150ml orange juice
1 mango, peeled and diced
2 teaspoons arrowroot

TIP *Allowing the duck to rest is important as it will continue to cook out of the pan and become more tender*

1 Preheat the oven to 200C, 400F, gas mark 6.
2 Prepare the duck by removing all the skin and visible fat with a sharp knife. Season each breast with cayenne pepper. Mix together the spices and parsley and rub on to the duck.
3 Heat a heavy-based, non-stick pan until hot. Add the duck and cook for 6–8 minutes on each side.
4 Meanwhile, heat the orange juice and mango in a saucepan. Mix the arrowroot with a little cold water to a paste and stir into the sauce to thicken it.
5 Remove the duck from the pan and allow to rest for 5 minutes.
6 Strain the meat juices from the duck into the fruit sauce.
7 Carve the duck and serve with the hot fruit sauce. Accompany with boiled basmati rice and a selection of fresh vegetables.

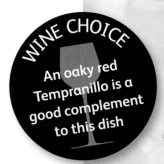

WINE CHOICE
An oaky red Tempranillo is a good complement to this dish

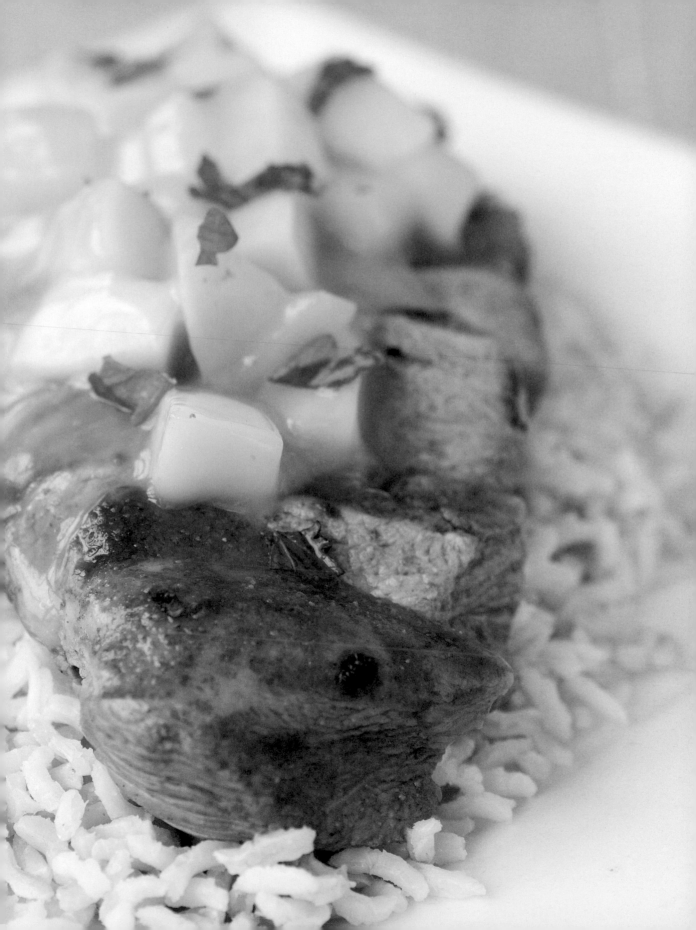

Rustic tomato chicken

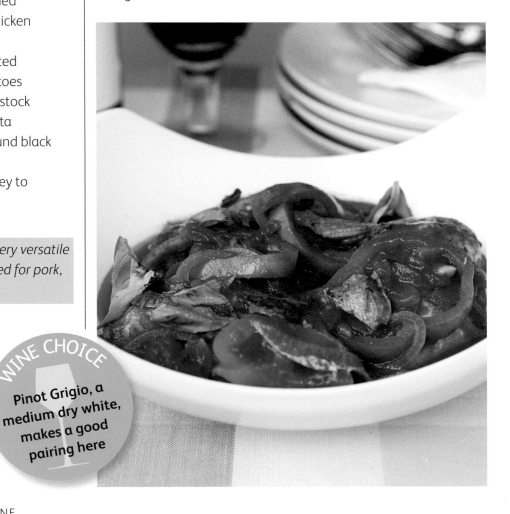

SERVES 4
PER SERVING
254 KCAL
5.7G FAT

PREPARATION TIME 5 MINUTES
COOKING TIME 30 MINUTES

2 red onions, chopped
2 garlic cloves, crushed
4 × 150g skinless chicken
 breasts
2 green peppers, sliced
1 × 400g can tomatoes
1 teaspoon chicken stock
500g tomato passata
salt and freshly ground black
 pepper
chopped fresh parsley to
 garnish

TIP *This sauce is very versatile and can also be used for pork, turkey and beef*

1 Heat a non-stick frying pan, and dry-fry the onion and garlic until soft.
2 Season the chicken breasts with salt and pepper and add to the pan, browning them on both sides. Add the peppers and continue cooking for 2–3 minutes.
3 Stir in the canned tomatoes, chicken stock and tomato passata. Simmer gently for 20 minutes until the chicken is fully cooked and the sauce reduced. Just before serving, sprinkle with the parsley.
4 Serve with boiled new potatoes (with skins) and green vegetables or salad

WINE CHOICE

Pinot Grigio, a medium dry white, makes a good pairing here

Beef steak and potato pie

1. Preheat the oven to 190C, 375F, gas mark 5.
2. Heat a heavy-based, non-stick pan, and dry-fry the beef until it changes colour. Drain through a metal sieve to remove as much fat as possible, and wipe out the pan with kitchen paper. Put the beef aside for a moment.
3. Add the onions and garlic to the pan and dry-fry for 2–3 minutes until soft.
4. Stir in the thyme, then return the beef to the pan. Add 2 tablespoons of beef stock and sprinkle the flour over. Mix well, cooking over a low heat for 1 minute, then gradually add the remaining stock. Add the swede and carrots, then simmer gently for 15 minutes to allow the mixture to thicken, stirring occasionally.
5. Stir in a little gravy browning for colour, if using, then transfer to an ovenproof dish.
6. Cover with layers of filo pastry, spraying lightly with oil spray in between each layer. Season well with black pepper and place in the oven for 20–25 minutes until golden brown. Garnish with fresh parsley and serve with a selection of fresh vegetables.

SERVES 4
PER SERVING
480 CALORIES
11.6G FAT

PREPARATION TIME 15 MINUTES
COOKING TIME 1 HOUR

500g lean beef steak, cubed
2 onions, finely chopped
1 garlic clove, crushed
2 teaspoons chopped fresh
   thyme
600ml beef stock
2 tablespoons plain flour
a little gravy browning
   (optional)
300g swede, peeled and diced
300g carrots, peeled and diced
4 sheets filo pastry
freshly ground black pepper
low-calorie oil spray
fresh parsley to garnish

TIP *You can make the base to this pie the day before, then, when ready to cook, simply top with filo pastry and bake in the oven*

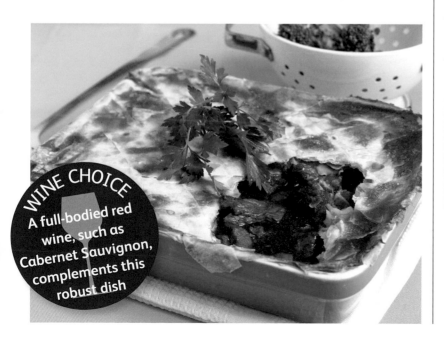

WINE CHOICE
A full-bodied red wine, such as Cabernet Sauvignon, complements this robust dish

Chicken enchiladas

SERVES 4
PER SERVING
430 CALORIES
6G FAT

PREPARATION TIME 10 MINUTES
COOKING TIME 35 MINUTES

450g minced chicken
2 red onions, finely chopped
2 garlic cloves, crushed
1–2 teaspoons chicken stock
   powder
1 fresh red chilli, chopped
2 red peppers, deseeded and
   finely sliced
1 tablespoon chopped fresh
   oregano, plus extra to
   garnish
1 × 400g can chopped
   tomatoes
500g tomato passata
300ml semi-skimmed milk
3 teaspoons cornflour
1 teaspoon Dijon mustard
4 flour tortillas
50g Rosemary Conley mature
   cheese, grated

TIP *You can buy vacuumed-packed tortillas with a long shelf life*

1 Preheat the oven to 200C, 400F, gas mark 6.
2 Heat a heavy-based, non-stick pan, and dry-fry the chicken until lightly browed. Add the onions and garlic and dry-fry for 2–3 minutes until soft.
3 Add the stock powder, chilli, peppers, oregano, chopped tomatoes and tomato passata. Simmer gently for 20–25 minutes until the sauce has thickened and the meat is tender.
4 In a separate pan, heat the milk. Slake the cornflour with a little cold water and whisk into the milk. Stir in the mustard as the sauce thickens.
5 Take one tortilla and place a line of chicken mixture down the centre. Roll up and place in an ovenproof dish. Repeat with the remaining tortillas, spoon some chicken mix over each enchilada. Pour the sauce over and sprinkle with grated cheese.
6 Bake in the oven for 20–25 minutes until golden brown.
7 Sprinkle some fresh oregano on top and serve with low-fat red pepper salsa and mixed salad leaves.

WINE CHOICE
Go for Pinot Grigio or be bold and try a hearty red Zinfandel

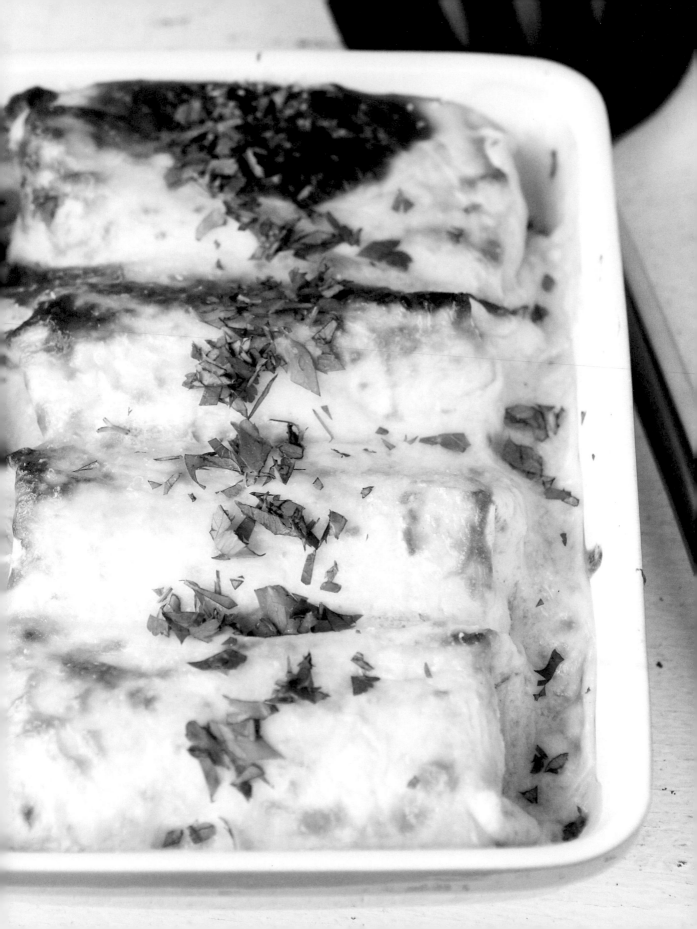

Wine marinated lamb

SERVES 4
PER SERVING
416 CALORIES
17.2G FAT

PREPARATION TIME 15 MINUTES
MARINATING TIME 20 MINUTES
COOKING TIME 15 MINUTES

1 tablespoon green
  peppercorns
900g lean lamb fillet, all visible
  fat removed
1 teaspoon chopped fresh
  thyme
1 tablespoon chopped fresh
  parsley
2 garlic cloves, finely chopped
300ml red wine
300ml water
1 teaspoon stock powder
1 tablespoon cornflour
1–2 drops gravy browning

TIP *Allow at least 20 minutes for the lamb to marinate as this will add flavour as well as tenderise the meat*

1 Crush the peppercorns, either in a pestle and mortar or put them on a chopping board and crush with the broad edge of a heavy chopping knife. Place the crushed peppercorns on a flat plate.

2 Dip the lamb into the peppercorns, pressing the peppercorns well into the meat. Sprinkle with the herbs and garlic and pour the red wine over. Leave to marinate for 20 minutes to allow the flavours to develop.

3 Preheat a conventional grill to high or preheat a contact health grill.

5 Lift the lamb from the marinade (reserve the marinade) and either put on to a non-stick baking tray and cook under the hot grill or place in the health grill. Grill for 2–3 minutes each side for rare, 3–4 minutes for medium and 5–6 minutes for well done.

5 While the lamb is cooking, heat the marinade with the water and the stock powder. Slake the cornflour with a little extra cold water, and gradually add to the sauce, stirring continuously to prevent lumps forming. Simmer gently to allow the sauce to thicken. Add the gravy browning to give the sauce a rich colour.

6 Slice the lamb and serve with a selection of fresh vegetables. Serve the sauce separately.

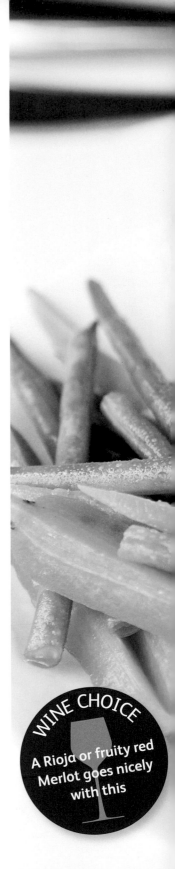

WINE CHOICE
A Rioja or fruity red Merlot goes nicely with this

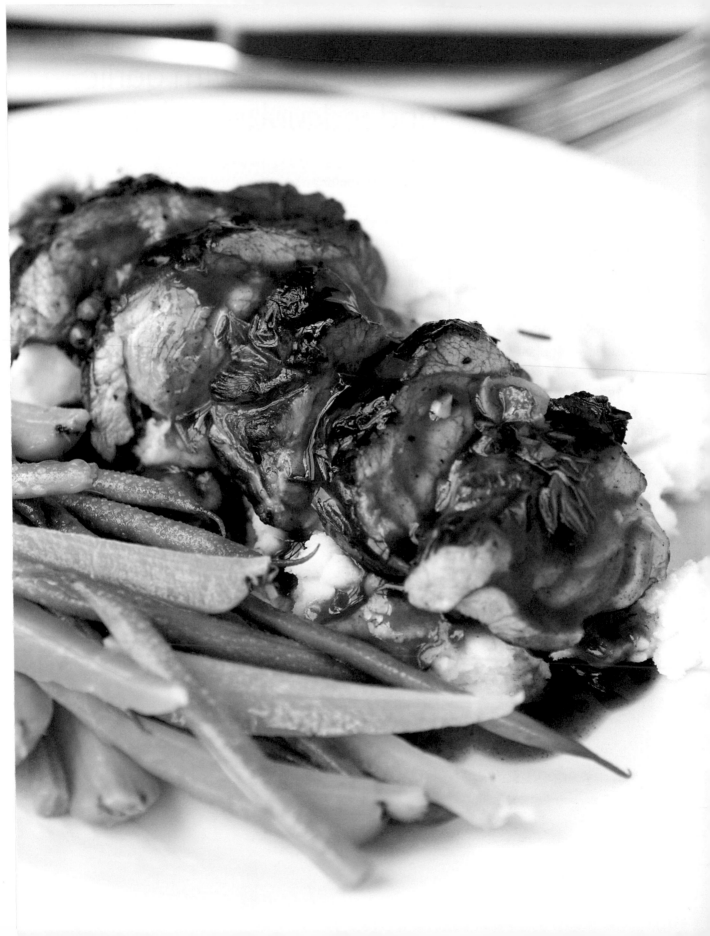

Mussels with white wine and spinach

SERVES 4
PER SERVING
311 CALORIES
6.3G FAT

PREPARATION TIME 15 MINUTES
COOKING TIME 10 MINUTES

1kg fresh mussels
1 onion, finely diced
2 garlic cloves, crushed
300ml dry white wine,
1–2 teaspoons vegetable stock
   powder
225g spinach, washed
1 tablespoon Alpro soya
   alternative to single cream
freshly ground black pepper

TIP *The Alpro soya makes this a dairy-free option. Be careful not to overcook the mussels – they only take a minute or so*

1 To clean the mussels, put them in a large bowl and scrape well under cold running water. Pull away the beard on the sides and discard any mussels that are open. Rinse until there is no trace of sand in the bowl.

2 Heat a large, non-stick saucepan, and gently dry-fry the onion for 3–4 minutes. Add the garlic and white wine and cook for a further 3–4 minutes.

3 Stir the stock powder into the pan, and add the mussels. Put the washed spinach on top, cover with a lid, and cook for 1–2 minutes, until the mussel shells open. Add the Alpro soya and stir well, seasoning with black pepper. Discard any mussels that do not open. Ladle the mussels into a bowl and serve at once.

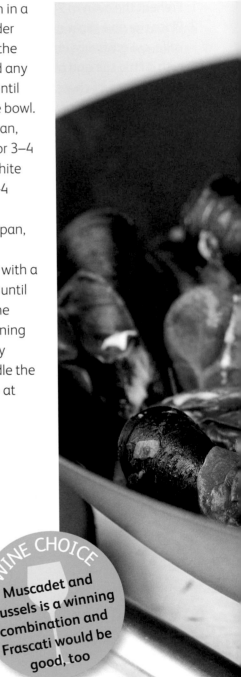

WINE CHOICE
Muscadet and mussels is a winning combination and Frascati would be good, too

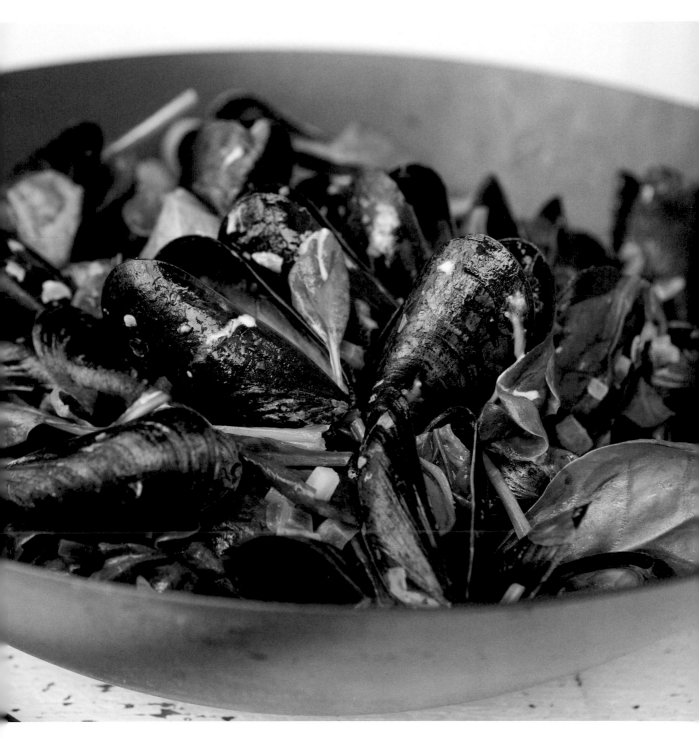

Baked smoked haddock with peppers

SERVES 4
PER SERVING
272 CALORIES
2.6G FAT

PREPARATION TIME 15 MINUTES
COOKING TIME 25 MINUTES

900g thick smoked haddock,
 skinned and cut into 4 steaks
1 red onion, finely chopped
1 garlic clove, crushed
1 long red pepper, deseeded
 and finely diced
1 × 400g can chopped
 tomatoes
1–2 teaspoons chilli sauce
1 tablespoon chopped fresh
 basil
juice of ½ lime
freshly ground black pepper

TIP *Choose thick pieces of haddock so they retain their moisture during cooking*

1 Preheat the oven to 200C, 400F, gas mark 6.
2 Season the fish on both sides with black pepper and place on a non-stick baking tray.
3 Heat a heavy-based, non-stick pan, and dry-fry the onion until soft. Add the garlic and red pepper, and cook until soft. Add the tomatoes and cook briskly for 4–5 minutes, stirring in the chilli sauce and basil. Add the lime juice, then remove from the heat.
4 Spoon equal amounts of the mixture on to each haddock steak and place, uncovered, in the hot oven for 12–15 minutes or until just cooked. Serve with green salad or vegetables.

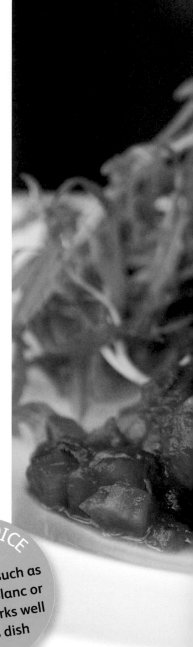

WINE CHOICE
A dry white, such as Sauvignon Blanc or Frascati, works well with this dish

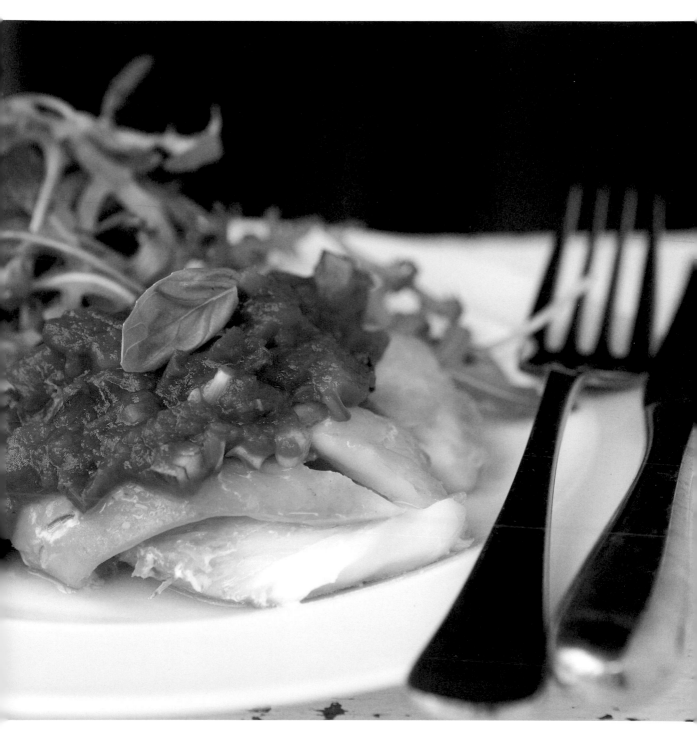

Salmon and sweet potato fishcakes

SERVES 4
PER SERVING
506 CALORIES
19.6G FAT

PREPARATION TIME 10 MINUTES
COOKING TIME 30 MINUTES

450g sweet potatoes, peeled
400g fresh salmon fillet
1 lime, sliced
4 baby leeks, finely sliced
1 tablespoon chopped fresh
    parsley
1 tablespoon chopped fresh
    chives
1 tablespoon grainy mustard
50g fresh granary breadcrumbs
salt and freshly ground black
    pepper

for the sauce
300ml semi-skimmed milk
1–2 teaspoons vegetable stock
    powder
4 teaspoons cornflour
2 teaspoons basil paste
2 teaspoons mild Dijon mustard

TIP *Drain the potatoes well,
as sweet potatoes retain more
water than ordinary ones*

1 Boil the potatoes in a large pan of water
   until soft. Drain and mash well and
   transfer to a large mixing bowl.
2 Place the salmon and lime in a saucepan.
   Cover with water and poach gently for 10
   minutes until cooked through. Drain and
   allow to cool.
3 Heat a non-stick frying pan, and dry-fry
   the leeks for 3–4 minutes until soft. Add to
   the potatoes and season with salt and
   black pepper. Mix in the herbs and the
   mustard.
4 Carefully flake the salmon into the potato
   mixture, removing any skin and bones.
   Mix the ingredients together, taking care
   not to break down the salmon.
5 Divide the mixture into 8 and shape into
   fishcakes with a palette knife. Spread out
   the granary breadcrumbs on a plate. Press
   the fishcakes into the breadcrumbs,
   coating all sides.
6 To make the sauce, heat the milk and
   stock powder in a small saucepan. Slake
   the cornflour with a little cold milk and
   whisk into the hot milk. Add the basil
   paste and mustard and simmer gently for
   5 minutes stirring continuously.
7 Heat a non-stick frying pan, and dry-fry
   the fishcakes for 8–10 minutes on each
   side. Transfer to a serving plate and
   spoon the sauce over. Serve hot with
   salad.

WINE CHOICE
Chablis is a classic
combination with
salmon but any
good, dry white
would suit

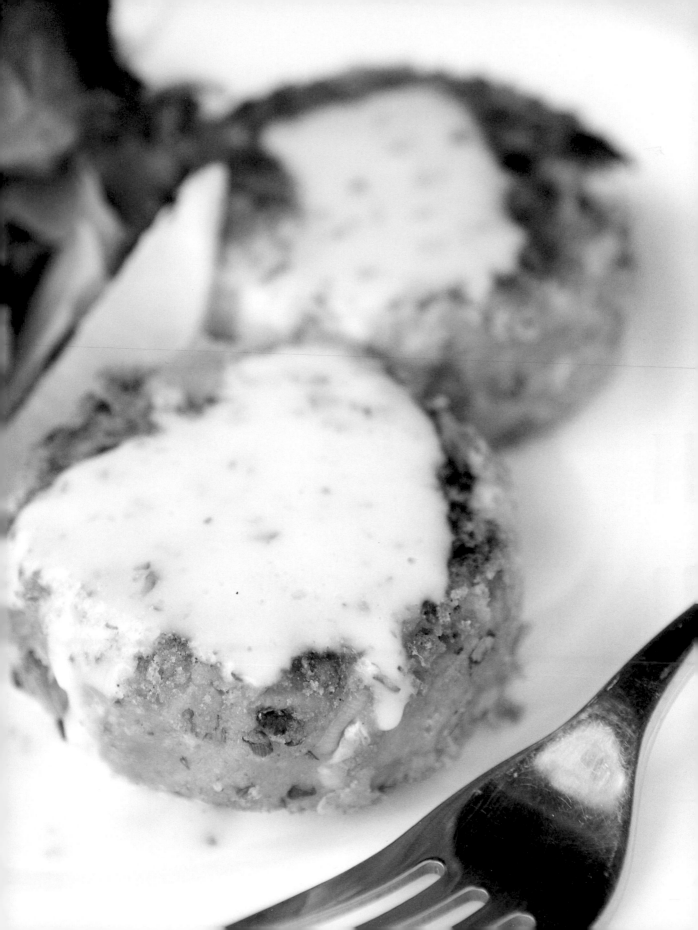

Spinach and ricotta pie

PER SERVING
SERVES 4
147 CALORIES
2G FAT

PREPARATION TIME 20 MINUTES
COOKING TIME 40 MINUTES

225g fresh baby spinach
1 garlic clove, crushed
225g ricotta cheese
pinch of nutmeg
2 teaspoons lemon zest
8 sheets filo pastry
low-calorie oil spray
salt and freshly ground black
    pepper

TIP *As an alternative, leave to cool, then cut the pie into squares and serve as a starter or as part of a buffet*

1 Preheat the oven to 200C, 400F, gas mark 6. Lightly grease a small non-stick-baking dish.
2 Using a large chopping knife, finely shred the spinach and place in a non-stick pan along with the garlic. Cook over a low heat until the spinach has wilted and reduced, then remove from the heat and allow to cool. Fold in the ricotta cheese, nutmeg and lemon zest, seasoning with salt and black pepper.
3 Take 1 sheet of filo pastry and use to line the baking dish, letting the pastry hang over the edges of the dish. Lightly spray with oil, then repeat with 3 more sheets. Pile the cheese and spinach mixture on top, then layer the remaining pastry sheets on top, folding the sides in with each layer.
4 Lightly spray the pastry topping with oil and place the dish near the bottom of the oven. Bake for 15–20 minutes until golden brown.
5 Serve hot with salad and steamed couscous.

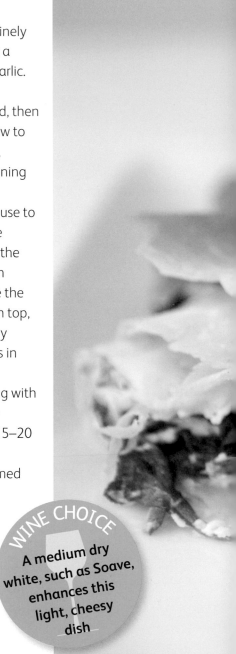

WINE CHOICE

A medium dry white, such as Soave, enhances this light, cheesy dish

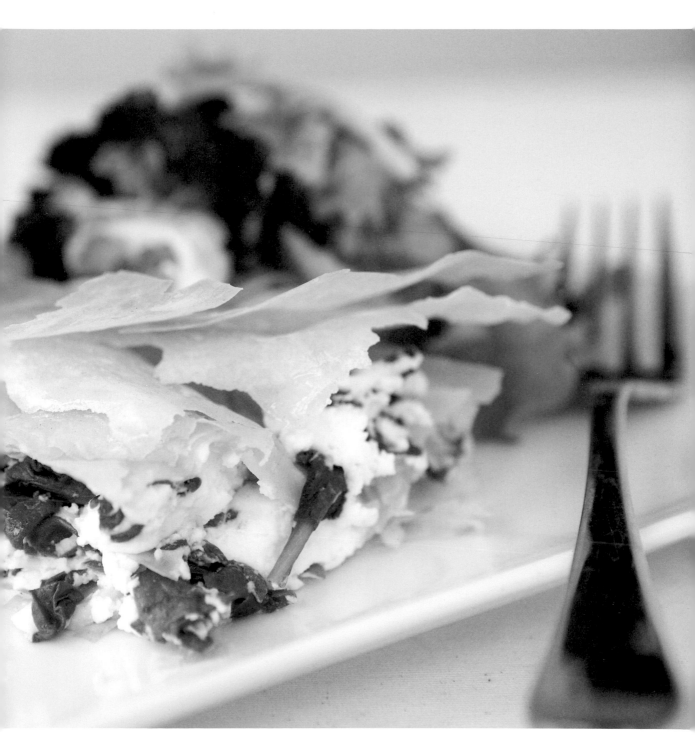

Paella

SERVES 4
PER SERVING
419 CALORIES
8.6G FAT

PREPARATION TIME 15 MINUTES
COOKING TIME 20 MINUTES

2 good pinches saffron strands
2 skinless chicken breasts, cubed
1 large onion, finely diced
2 garlic cloves, crushed
225g Arborio risotto rice
600ml vegetable stock
450g prepared seafood (e.g.
    squid, octopus, prawns)
225g cod fillet
115g frozen peas
450g cleaned mussels
freshly ground black pepper
lemon wedges to garnish

TIP *If you don't have a pan big enough to accommodate everything, cook the mussels in a separate pan in a little vegetable stock and add to the finished dish*

1 Infuse the saffron strands in a little boiling water for 5 minutes.
2 Heat a large, non-stick frying pan and dry-fry the chicken until lightly coloured. Remove from the pan and set aside.
3 Add the onion and garlic to the pan and dry-fry until soft.
4 Add the rice, vegetable stock and infused saffron to the pan, stirring well. Bring to a gentle simmer for 10 minutes, then add the chicken and continue cooking until the rice is almost done.
5 Add the prepared seafood, cod and frozen peas, and stir well. Add a little more stock if all the existing stock has been absorbed.
6 Arrange the mussels on top and cover with a lid. Cook for 4–5 minutes until all the mussels have opened.
7 Sprinkle with freshly ground black pepper, garnish with lemon wedges and serve immediately.

WINE CHOICE
A crisp, dry white, such as Chablis, is the perfect pairing for paella

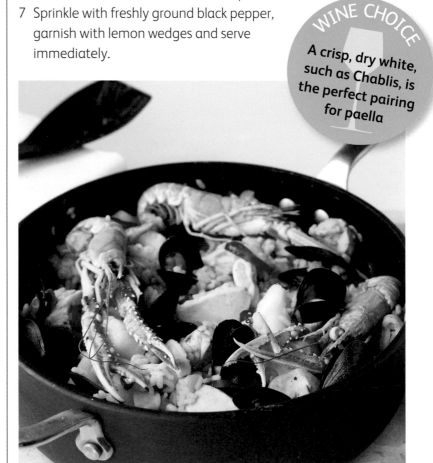

Veggie cottage pie

1 Preheat the oven to 200C, 400F, gas mark 6. Cook the potatoes in boiling water with the stock cube, adding the leeks 5 minutes before the end of cooking.
2 Meanwhile, heat a non-stick frying pan, and dry-fry the Quorn mince, onion and garlic for 3–4 minutes, stirring in the stock powder during cooking.
3 Add the carrots, tomato passata, vegetable stock and herbs and simmer gently for 20 minutes to let the sauce thicken. Season with black pepper and transfer to an ovenproof dish.
4 Drain the potatoes and leeks then mash well, adding skimmed milk and half the cheese. Season with black pepper.
5 Spread the potato mixture over the Quorn and smooth over with a fork. Sprinkle with the remaining cheese and place on the top shelf of the oven for 20 minutes until golden brown.
6 Serve with steamed green vegetables.

SERVES 4
PER SERVING
346 CALORIES
7.7G FAT

PREPARATION TIME 10 MINUTES
COOKING TIME 40 MINUTES

675g potatoes, chopped
1 vegetable stock cube
2 leeks, sliced
1 × 450g pack Quorn mince
1 red onion, chopped
2 garlic cloves, crushed
2 teaspoons vegetable bouillon
    stock powder
3 carrots, diced
600ml tomato passata
300ml vegetable stock
1 tablespoon chopped herbs
    (e.g. oregano, parsley,
    thyme)
2 tablespoons skimmed milk
50g low-fat vegetarian cheddar-
    style cheese, grated
freshly ground black pepper

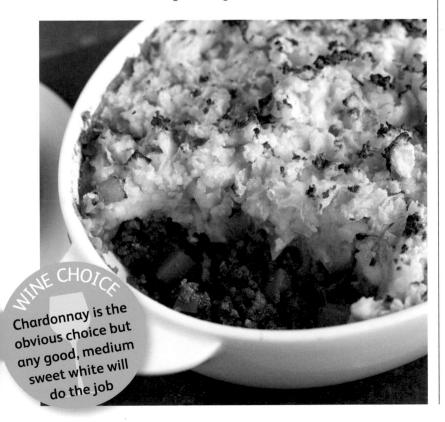

WINE CHOICE
Chardonnay is the obvious choice but any good, medium sweet white will do the job

TIP *You can freeze Quorn mince and use it straight from the freezer*

Sweet potato and fennel gratin

SERVES 4
PER SERVING
304 CALORIES
3.7G FAT

PREPARATION TIME 20 MINUTES
COOKING TIME 65 MINUTES

900g sweet potatoes, peeled
1 bulb fennel, finely sliced
1 medium onion, finely sliced
1 garlic clove, crushed
a little grated fresh nutmeg
2 teaspoons vegetable bouillon
    stock powder
50g low-fat vegetarian cheddar-
    style cheese, grated
600ml skimmed milk
freshly ground black pepper
1 tablespoon chopped fresh
    parsley to garnish

TIP *As sweet potatoes do not
discolour, they can be peeled
in advance*

1. Preheat the oven to 200C, 400F, gas mark 6.
2. Thinly slice the potatoes into a large bowl. Add the fennel, onion and garlic along with the nutmeg and some black pepper. Stir in the stock powder and mix together well. Layer into a lightly greased ovenproof dish and cover with the grated cheese.
3. Heat the milk in a saucepan, then pour it over the potatoes. Bake in the centre of the oven for 60 minutes until soft. Serve straight away sprinkled with chopped parsley.

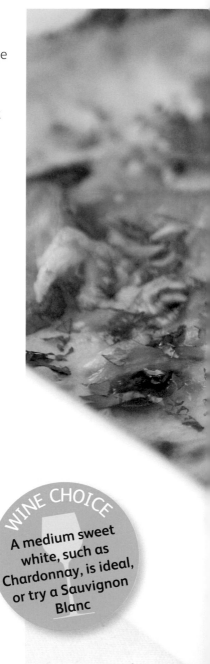

WINE CHOICE
A medium sweet white, such as Chardonnay, is ideal, or try a Sauvignon Blanc

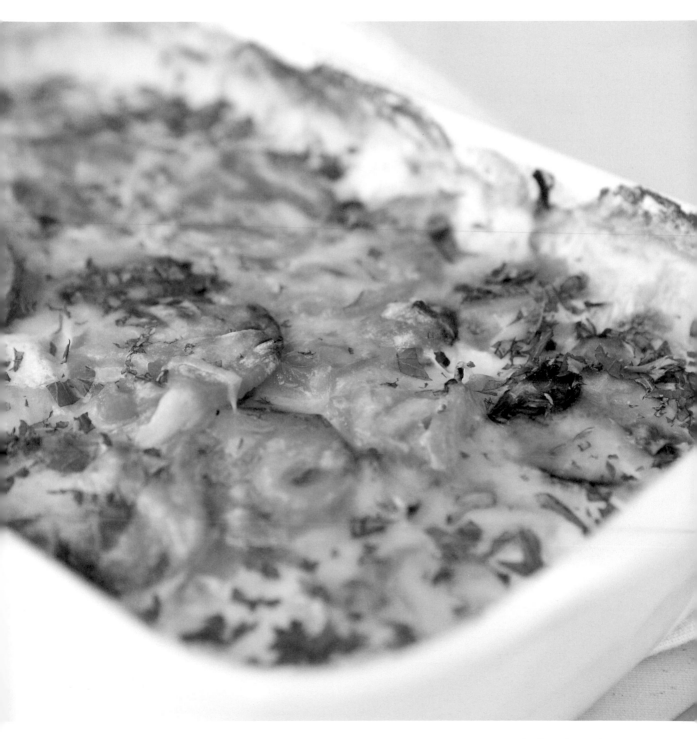

Crunchy topped broccoli and cauliflower cheese

SERVES 4
PER SERVING
261 CALORIES
8.6G FAT

PREPARATION TIME 5 MINUTES
COOKING TIME 25–28 MINUTES

225g fresh broccoli
225g fresh cauliflower
2 onions, cut into quarters
1 vegetable stock cube
600ml semi-skimmed milk
1 teaspoon vegetable stock
  powder
1 tablespoon arrowroot
2 teaspoons Dijon mustard
100g low-fat vegetarian hard
  cheese, grated
10g fresh breadcrumbs
1 tablespoon chopped chives
freshly ground black pepper

TIP *For a more substantial meal, place some mashed sweet potatoes in the base of the dish before adding the vegetables and sauce*

1 Preheat the oven to 200C, 400F, gas mark 6.
2 Cut the broccoli and cauliflower into florets. Cook in a shallow pan of boiling water containing the onions and stock cube for 5–8 minutes. Drain well and transfer to an ovenproof dish.
3 Heat the milk to near boiling. Mix the arrowroot with a little extra cold water and whisk into the hot milk along with the mustard and half the cheese. Simmer the sauce until thickened, then pour over the vegetables.
4 Mix the remaining cheese with the breadcrumbs and chives, season with black pepper and sprinkle over the sauce.
5 Bake in the oven for 20 minutes until brown and toasted on top.

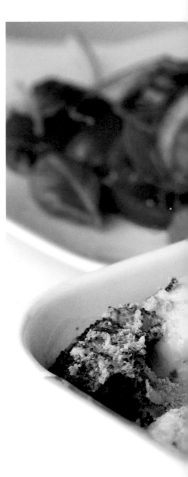

WINE CHOICE
You won't go wrong with a good Chardonnay, or other medium white

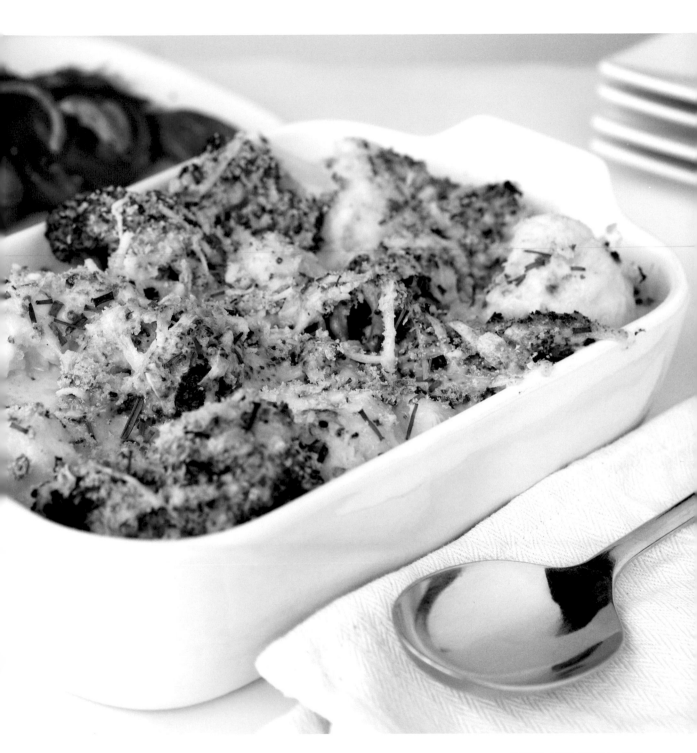

Quorn potato bake

SERVES 4
PER SERVING
323 CALORIES
5.2G FAT

PREPARATION TIME 15 MINUTES
COOKING TIME 50 MINUTES

1 red onion, diced
2 garlic cloves, crushed
1 × 312g pack plain Quorn
   fillets
2 celery sticks, chopped
1 tablespoon flour
125ml white wine
1 tablespoon chopped fresh
   tarragon
2 teaspoons vegetable stock
   powder, plus 1 teaspoon
450ml semi-skimmed milk
4 large red potatoes
chopped fresh parsley to
   garnish

TIP *Quorn fillets can be cut into pieces and used in casseroles and curries*

1 Preheat the oven to 200C, 400F, gas mark 6.
2 Heat a non-stick frying pan, and dry-fry the onion and garlic until soft. Add the Quorn fillets and celery. Sprinkle the flour over the fillets and cook out for 1 minute.
3 Stir in the wine. Add the tarragon and 2 teaspoons of stock powder and gradually stir in the milk. Simmer gently to allow the sauce to thicken while you cook the potatoes.
4 Peel and slice the potatoes and place in a saucepan. Cover with boiling water and add the remaining teaspoon of stock powder. Boil until the potatoes are soft, and then drain them.
5 Spoon the Quorn mixture into the bottom of an ovenproof dish and top with the sliced potatoes.
6 Bake in the oven for 25 minutes until golden brown.
7 Remove from the oven, sprinkle with parsley and serve with an assortment of fresh vegetables.

WINE CHOICE
Chardonnay works well here, or try Pinot Blanc or Chablis

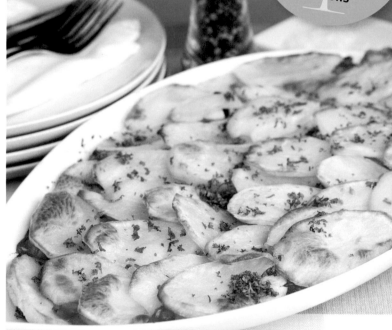

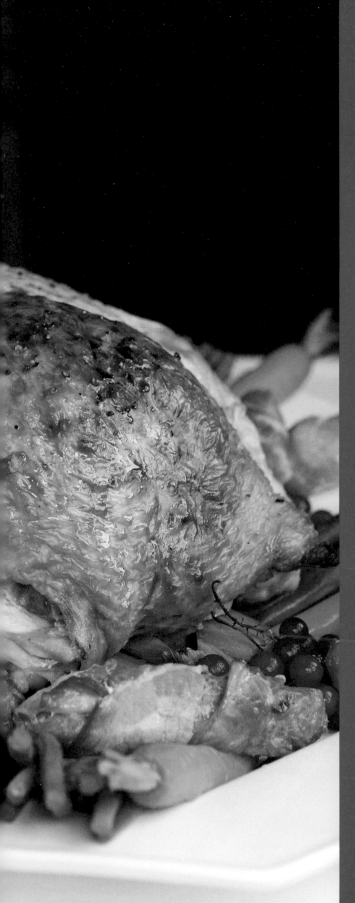

Have a low-fat Christmas

Serve up these fabulously tasty Christmas dishes and your family and friends will never guess they're low in fat. Here, you'll find mouthwatering meat and vegetarian options for a traditional festive lunch as well as recipes for Christmas pudding, meringue-topped mince pies and, of course, a low Gi Christmas cake. And don't forget to put the champagne on ice!

Melon and prawn cocktail

SERVES 6 AS A STARTER
PER SERVING
42 CALORIES
0.5G FAT

PREPARATION TIME 10 MINUTES

1 cantaloupe melon
1 × 105g pack cooked king
    prawns
a few fresh rocket leaves
4 lemon slices to garnish

for the sauce
2 tablespoons extra light
    mayonnaise
1 tablespoon tomato ketchup
dash of chilli sauce
lemon juice to taste

TIP *If you don't have a melon baller, use a serrated knife and cut the melon into cubes*

1 Cut the melon half and remove the seeds. Using a melon baller, remove the flesh and set aside.
2 Shred the rocket leaves and place in the base of 4 glasses or dishes. Add the melon balls and cooked prawns, reserving 4 prawns for the garnish.
3 Mix together the sauce ingredients and spoon on top.
4 Garnish each glass with a reserved prawn and a slice of lemon.

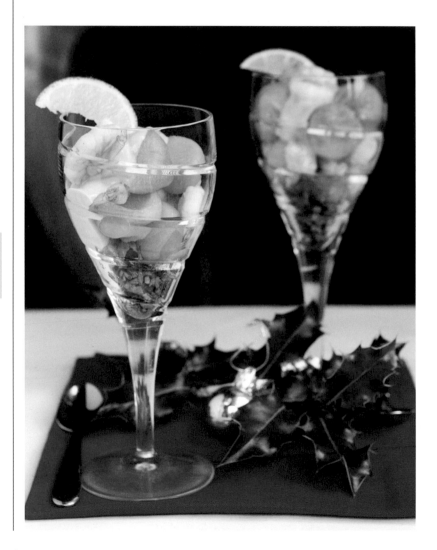

Scallops with lime and coriander

1 Rinse the scallops well and place on kitchen paper to dry.
2 In a bowl, mix the ginger with a little salt and pepper. Roll the scallops in the seasoning.
3 Arrange the salad leaves on serving plates.
4 Heat a non-stick frying pan and lightly spray with olive oil spray. Add the scallops and cook quickly for 1 minute on each side.
5 Squeeze the lime juice over the scallops and sprinkle with the coriander. Remove from the heat and arrange on top of the salad leaves. Serve straight away.

SERVES 4 AS A STARTER
PER SERVING
70 CALORIES
1.1G FAT

PREPARATION TIME 5 MINUTES
COOKING TIME 10 MINUTES

12 fresh scallops
1 × 2cm piece fresh ginger, peeled and finely chopped
a few salad leaves
coarse sea salt and black pepper
low-calorie olive oil spray
juice of ½ lime
1 tablespoon chopped fresh coriander to garnish

TIP *Cook the scallops at the last minute so they don't overcook and become tough*

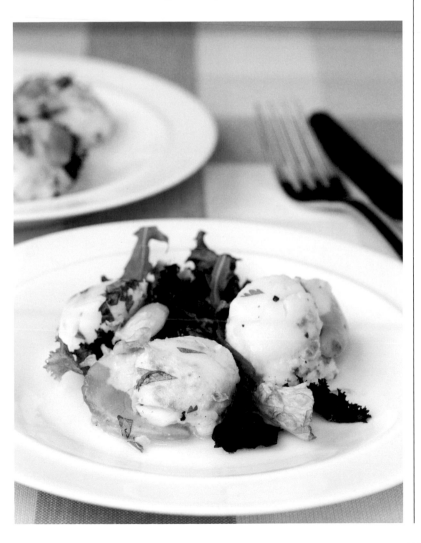

Roast turkey crown with leek and parsley stuffing

SERVES 6
PER SERVING
413 CALORIES
6.7G FAT

PREPARATION TIME 20 MINUTES
COOKING TIME 2–3 HOURS

1 × 1.8kg turkey crown
1 head celery
1 red onion, peeled
redcurrants to garnish

for the stuffing
2 leeks, finely chopped
100g granary breadcrumbs
100g Bowyers 95% fat-free
  sausages, chopped
2 tablespoons chopped fresh
  parsley
1 teaspoon vegetable stock
  powder

TIP *Sitting the turkey on a head of celery adds flavour and also stops the joint from moving around during cooking*

1 Make the stuffing by dry-frying the leeks in a preheated non-stick pan until soft. Spoon into a mixing bowl, then mix in the remaining ingredients, adding a little boiling water from a kettle. Put aside and leave to cool.
2 Weigh the turkey and calculate the cooking time from the instructions given (or allow 15 minutes per 450g plus an extra 20 minutes). Preheat the oven to 190C, 375F, gas mark 5.
3 Rinse the turkey well under running cold water and pat dry with kitchen paper. Place the prepared stuffing under the skin, then fold the skin over to keep the stuffing in place.
4 Place the head of celery on a wire rack and sit the turkey on top.
5 Cut the onion into wedges and arrange around the turkey.
6 Place the wire rack over the roasting tin and pour 600ml water into the tin, around the rack.
7 Cover with foil and roast in the oven, basting occasionally with the juices.
8 Remove the turkey from the oven and allow to rest for 5–15 minutes before carving.
9 Garnish with redcurrants and serve with a selection of side dishes (see pages 224–5).

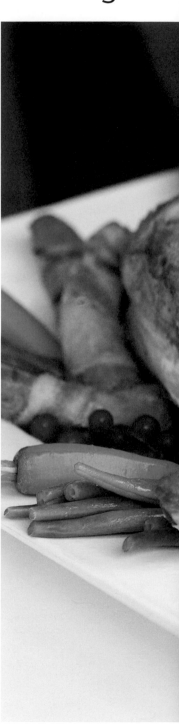

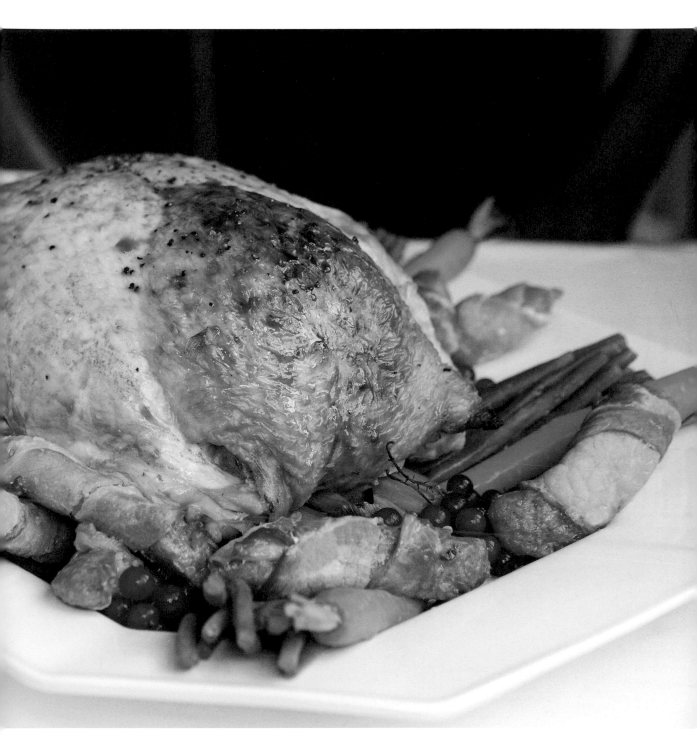

Low-fat gravy

Drain the meat juices from the turkey into a gravy separator. Allow the juices to stand and settle as the fat separates out. Then drain off the meat juices from the bottom of the gravy separator into a saucepan. Add more water (or vegetable stock) if required and thicken with a little gravy powder. Serve hot alongside the turkey.

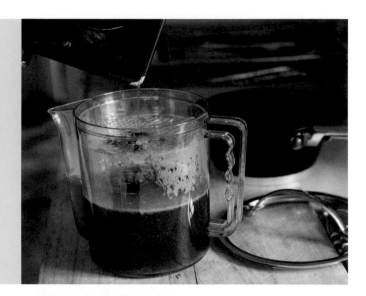

How to carve the turkey

Allow the roast joint to rest before carving for about 5–15 minutes, depending on its size. This allows the meat to reabsorb the juices released during cooking and give an even surface when sliced.

It's best to cut across the grain of the meat. The more tender the cut, the thicker the slices should be. Always carve with the blade of the knife facing away from you and use long cutting strokes the full length of the knife.

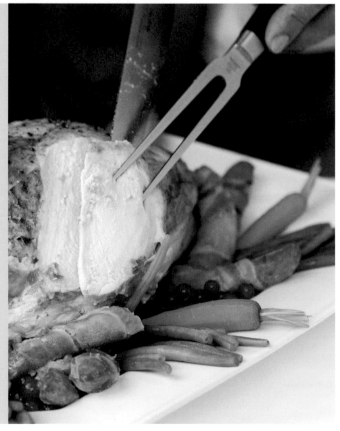

Aubergine crown Provençal

1 Preheat the oven to 200C, 400F, gas mark 6. Trim the tops and bottoms off both aubergines and cut each aubergine in half to give 4 barrel shapes.

2 Stand the barrels upright and cut a cross in the top of each one, pushing the knife halfway down each barrel. Repeat, cutting another cross in the top, so you end up with 8 sections.

3 Using a spoon, scoop out about two-thirds of the flesh from the centre of each barrel, and reserve.

4 Place the barrels upturned on a non-stick baking tray. Bake in the oven for 10–15 minutes until soft.

5 Chop the reserved aubergine flesh, and dry-fry in a hot, non-stick pan with the red onion, garlic and red pepper for 2–3 minutes. Add the diced courgettes and chopped mushrooms and continue cooking for 4–5 minutes. Stir in the herbs and chopped tomatoes and simmer for 5 minutes to reduce.

6 Remove the aubergine barrels from the oven. Turn them over and fill with the mixture. Return to the oven to heat through.

SERVES 4
PER SERVING
76 CALORIES
0.9G FAT

PREPARATION TIME 10 MINUTES
COOKING TIME 30 MINUTES

2 medium aubergines
1 red onion, chopped
1 garlic clove, crushed
1 red pepper, finely chopped
2 courgettes, diced
100g chestnut mushrooms, chopped
1 tablespoon chopped fresh herbs (e.g. basil, parsley, oregano)
1 × 400g can chopped tomatoes

TIP *You can make this vegetarian main course in advance and heat through just before serving*

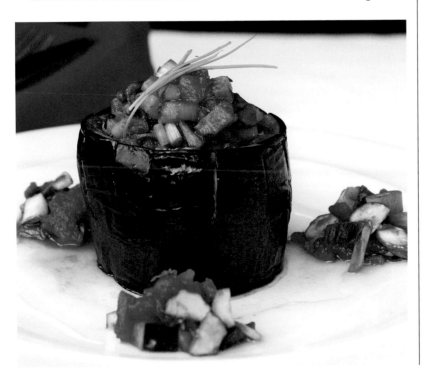

Bacon rolls

MAKES 12 ROLLS
PER ROLL
29 CALORIES
1.1G FAT

PREPARATION TIME 10 MINUTES
COOKING TIME 15–20 MINUTES

6 Bowyers 95 % fat free
   sausages
6 rashers plain or smoked back
   bacon

1 Preheat the oven to 200C, 400F, gas mark 6.
2 Using a sharp serrated knife, cut each sausage in half
   lengthways.
3 Using scissors, trim away the rind and any fat from the outside
   edges of the bacon and cut each slice in half lengthways.
4 Wrap the bacon around the sausages and place on a non-stick
   baking tray.
5 Cook in the oven for 15–20 minutes until lightly browned. Serve
   hot alongside the turkey.

Brussels sprouts with chestnuts ☑

SERVES 6
PER SERVING
78 CALORIES
2.1G FAT

PREPARATION TIME 15 MINUTES
COOKING TIME 15 MINUTES

600g brussels sprouts, loose
   outer leaves removed
1 vegetable stock cube
115g peeled and cooked
   chestnuts, chopped
grated fresh nutmeg
salt and freshly ground black
   pepper

1 Make a small nick in the stalk of each sprout. Cook in boiling
   water with the stock cube until just tender. Drain well and return
   to the pan.
2 Add the chestnuts and mix well. Season and sprinkle with
   nutmeg to taste.

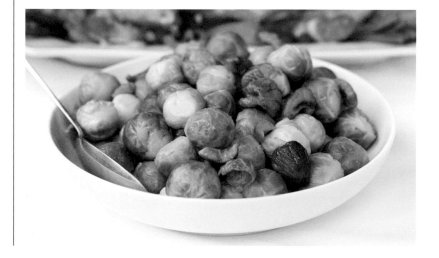

Roast parsnips and sweet potatoes

1 Preheat the oven to 200C, 400F, gas mark 6. Peel the vegetables and chop into equal-sized pieces.
2 Boil the parsnips and potatoes separately in water with the stock cubes until not quite fully cooked.
3 Drain the vegetables, reserving the liquid for the gravy stock, and place on a non-stick baking tray.
4 Spray the vegetables very lightly with olive oil spray and roast near the top of the oven until golden brown.

SERVES 6
PER SERVING
157 CALORIES
1.8G FAT

PREPARATION TIME 10 MINUTES
COOKING TIME 30 MINUTES

600g parsnips
600g sweet potatoes
2 vegetable stock cubes
salt and freshly ground black
    pepper
low-calorie olive oil spray

TIP *You can peel the sweet potatoes in advance as they do not discolour like regular ones*

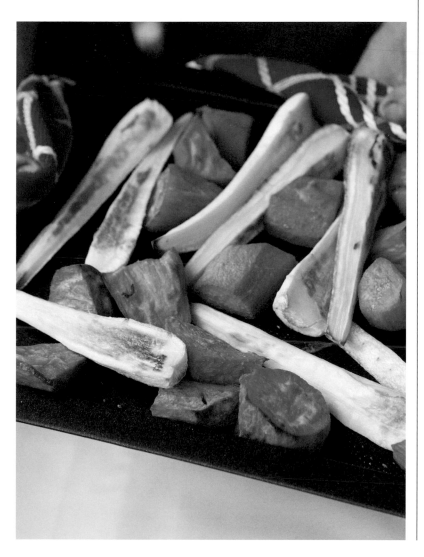

Low Gi Christmas pudding

SERVES 10
PER SERVING
197 CALORIES
1.7G FAT

PREPARATION TIME 20 MINUTES
COOKING TIME: STEAM 3 HOURS;
MICROWAVE 15 MINUTES

300g luxury mixed dried fruit
4 tablespoons brandy, rum or
   beer
75g plain flour
1 teaspoon mixed spice
½ teaspoon ground cinnamon
50g fresh granary breadcrumbs
50g dark brown sugar
2 teaspoons gravy browning
zest of ½ lemon
zest of ½ orange
100g grated cooking apple
100g grated carrot
1 tablespoon lemon juice
2 eggs, beaten
4 tablespoons skimmed milk
2 tablespoons molasses
4 tablespoons brandy for
   reheating

TIP *Soaking the fruit
overnight gives a rich, moist
pudding with lots of flavour*

1 Soak the dried fruit in the alcohol overnight. The next day, place the fruit in a large mixing bowl. Add the ingredients one at a time, mixing well.
2 Spoon the mixture into a 1.2 litre pudding basin.
3 Cook the pudding. To steam, cover with foil and steam gently for 3 hours. (To reheat, steam for 1–2 hours.) To microwave, cover with clingfilm and place an upturned plate on top, then cook on high speed for 5 minutes. Allow to stand for 5 minutes, then cook for a further 5 minutes. (To reheat, cook on high power for 5 minutes.)

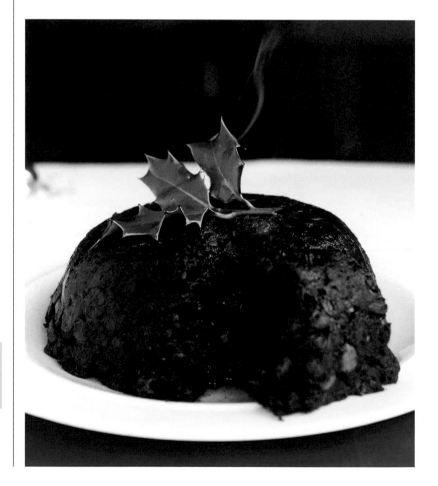

Meringue-topped mince pies

1 Preheat the oven to 190C, 375F, gas mark 5. Lightly grease a non-stick, 12-section mould with olive oil spray.
2 Stack the filo pastry sheets on top of each other and, using scissors, cut into 48 individual squares.
4 Put 4 squares into each mould section, placing the squares at slight angles to each other, and lightly spray with a fine mist of oil. Spoon the mincemeat into each pastry case.
5 For the topping, whisk the egg whites until stiff, then fold in the caster sugar. Spoon on top of the mince pies, swirling the meringue with a fork.
6 Bake in the centre of the oven for 10–15 minutes until crisp. Dust with icing sugar and serve warm.

MAKES 12
PER SERVING
93 CALORIES
1.7G FAT

PREPARATION TIME 20 MINUTES
COOKING TIME 20 MINUTES

4 sheets filo pastry
100g fat-free mincemeat
low-calorie olive oil spray

for the topping
2 egg whites
100g caster sugar
icing sugar to dust

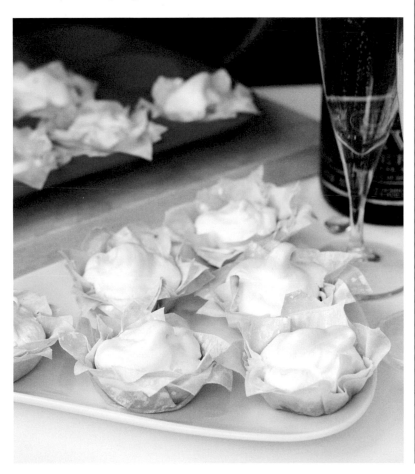

Low-fat Christmas cake

MAKES APPROX. 20 SLICES
PER SLICE
228 CALORIES
2.8G FAT

PREPARATION TIME 30 MINUTES
COOKING TIME 2–2½ HOURS

225g no pre-soak prunes, pitted
115g cooking apple, grated
175g dark muscovado sugar
4 eggs, beaten
zest of 1 lemon and 1 orange
175g self-raising flour, sifted
1 tablespoon mixed spice
50g sunflower seeds
225g currants
225g sultanas
225g raisins
115g glacé cherries
120ml brandy
2 tablespoons apricot jam, to
    glaze

TIP *This cake is best made a week in advance and stored in an airtight container*

1 Preheat the oven to 170C, 325F, gas mark 3. Line a cake tin (20cm × 7.5cm deep) with parchment paper.
2 In a large mixing bowl mix together the prunes and apple. Add the sugar, then beat in the eggs a little at a time. Press down to squash the prunes.
3 Mix in the lemon and orange zest, then carefully fold in the flour, spice, sunflower seeds and dried fruit.
4 Gradually stir in the brandy, then pour into the prepared cake tin.
5 Using the back of a metal spoon, make a slight dip in the centre to allow for an even top once baked. Bake for 2–2½ hours or until a metal skewer inserted into the cake comes out clean. Cool on a wire rack. Remove the parchment paper and brush with warmed apricot jam.

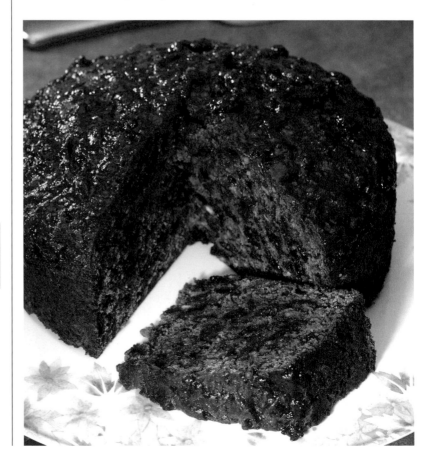

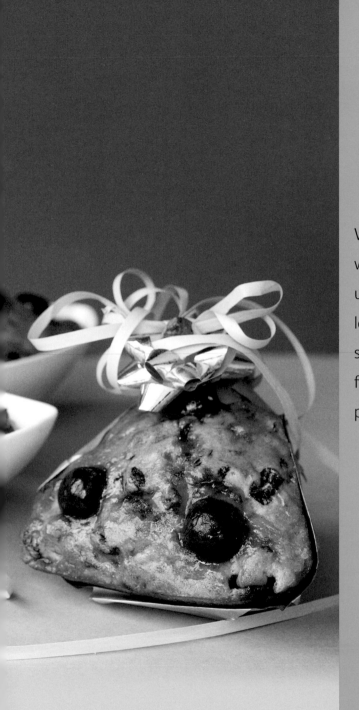

Party food

When it's party time, you're likely to want to lay out a special spread but the usual buffet-style offerings are often laden with fat and calories. So here are some scrumptious suggestions for low-fat finger or fork food that will make your party go with a swing!

Alan's beef fajitas

MAKES 12
PER FAJITA (TORTILLA AND FILLING)
195 CALORIES
4.1G FAT

PREPARATION TIME 10 MINUTES
COOKING TIME 10 MINUTES

1 red onion, chopped
1 garlic clove, crushed
3 lean rump steaks (350g total),
    cut into strips
sprig of fresh thyme
1 tablespoon soy sauce
1 red pepper, deseeded and
    diced
1 green pepper, deseeded and
    diced
1–2 tablespoons fajita spice mix
2 tablespoons plum tomatoes,
    blended

for serving
12 corn tortillas
2 extras per fajita (see above
    choices)

extras

2 teaspoons Discovery Mexican
sour cream
    20 CALORIES
    0.4G FAT

2 teaspoons low-fat guacamole
    20 CALORIES
    1.5G FAT

1–2 sliced jalapeño peppers
    PER JALAPEÑO
    2 CALORIES
    0.01G FAT

2 teaspoons grated Rosemary Conley
mature cheese
    PER 2 TEASPOONS
    19 CALORIES
    0.5G FAT

1 Heat a non-stick frying pan, and
   dry-fry the onion and garlic until
   soft. Add the beef and thyme and
   cook for 1–2 minutes, drizzling with
   soy sauce.
2 Add the peppers and fajita mix, and
   stir well to coat with the spices.
   Once the beef has changed colour,
   add the blended tomatoes and
   heat through until the beef is
   cooked to your liking.
3 Spoon a twelfth of the beef and
   tomato mixture on to each tortilla,
   add 2 extras of your choice to each
   one. Roll them up and serve.

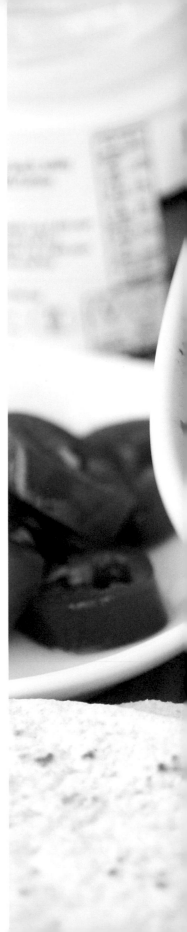

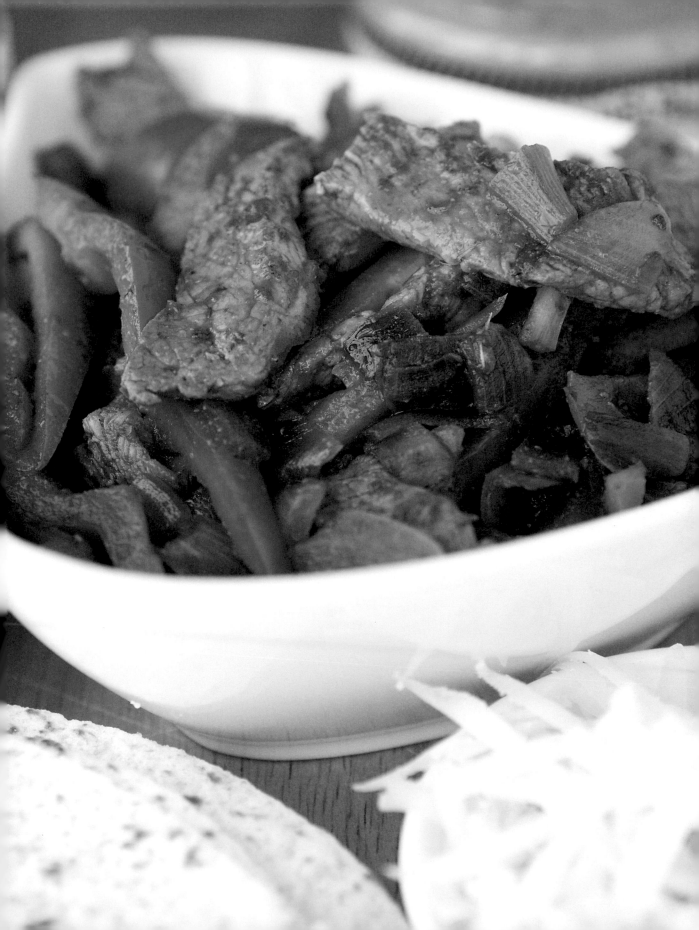

Tandoori chicken drumsticks

SERVES 4
PER SERVING
186 CALORIES
5G FAT

PREPARATION TIME 10 MINUTES
MARINATING TIME 30 MINUTES
COOKING TIME 35 MINUTES

8 × 47g fresh chicken
    drumsticks
2 garlic cloves, crushed
1 tablespoon tandoori powder
2 teaspoons ground coriander
300ml 3 % fat-yogurt
1 teaspoon ground ginger
salt and freshly ground black
    pepper

TIP *Removing the skin from the drumsticks not only reduces the fat content but also allows the spices to penetrate the meat*

1 Preheat the oven to 200C, 400F, gas mark 6.
2 Pull away the skin from the chicken drumsticks and discard.
3 Mix the spices with the garlic and yogurt and place in a shallow dish. Press the chicken into mixture, coating all sides. Allow to marinate for 30 minutes.
4 Transfer the chicken to a non-stick baking tray and place in a hot oven for 30 minutes until fully cooked.

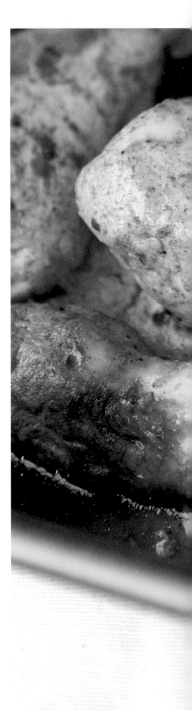

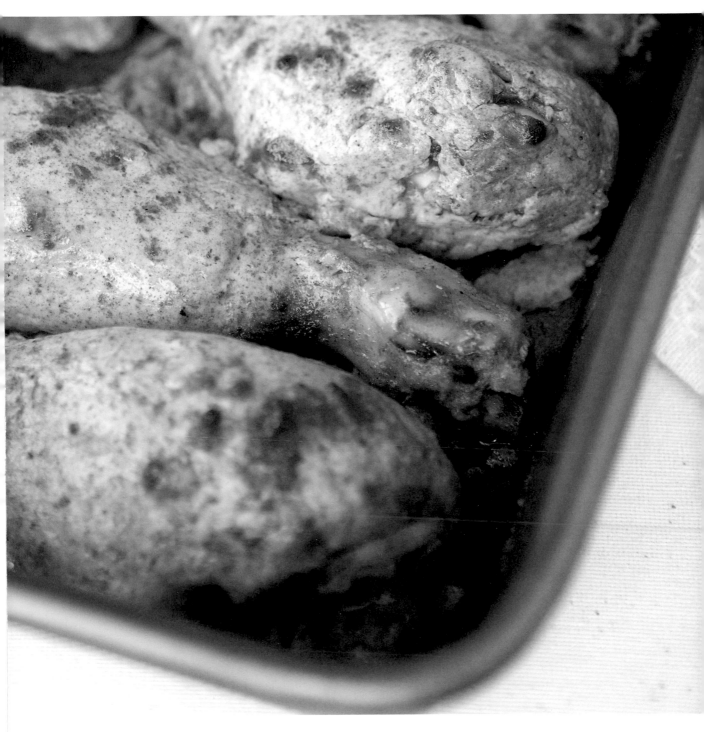

Debra's honey roast peppers

MAKES 16 PIECES
PER PEPPER QUARTER
17 CALORIES
0.2G FAT

PREPARATION TIME 10 MINUTES
COOKING TIME 20 MINUTES

2 red peppers
2 yellow peppers
8 cherry tomatoes
1 garlic clove, finely chopped
1 tablespoon runny honey
freshly ground black pepper
16 basil leaves

TIP *Once the peppers are cooked, spike each quarter with a cocktail stick to make them easier to handle*

1 Preheat the oven to 200C, 400F, gas mark 6.
2 Cut the peppers into quarters, remove the seeds and place the pepper quarters on a non-stick baking tray.
3 Cut the cherry tomatoes in half and place a half tomato in each pepper quarter. Sprinkle with chopped garlic and black pepper. Drizzle the honey over and bake in the oven for 15–20 minutes.
4 When cooked, allow to cool and garnish each pepper quarter with a basil leaf.

Debra's honey roast peppers and mini corn scones

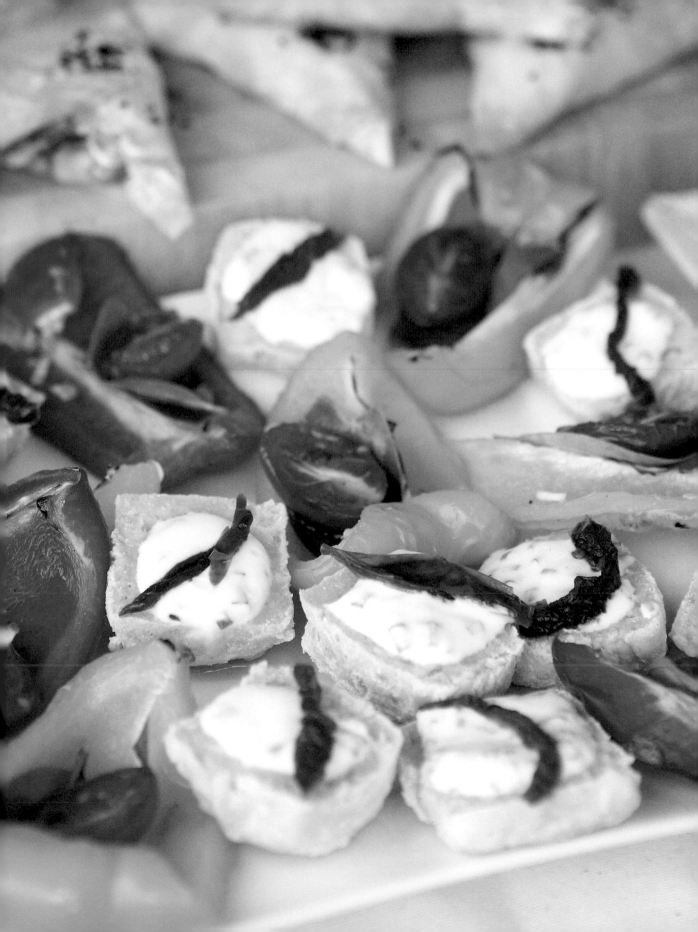

Debra's mini corn scones

MAKES 24 MINI SCONES
PER MINI (HALF) SCONE
42 CALORIES
0.5G FAT

PREPARATION TIME 15 MINUTES
COOKING TIME 20 MINUTES

180g plain flour
60g fine cornmeal
1 teaspoon baking powder
pinch of salt
2 tablespoons low-fat yogurt
150ml semi-skimmed milk

for the topping
2 sun-dried tomatoes, soaked
1 tablespoon low-fat yogurt
1 tablespoon finely chopped
    chives
freshly ground black pepper

TIP *You can also use homemade pesto or canned fish mixed with horseradish sauce for the topping*

1 Preheat the oven to 200C, 400F, gas mark 6.
2 In a mixing bowl combine the dry ingredients with the yogurt. Using a knife, bring the mixture together, gradually adding the milk until a soft dry dough is achieved.
3 Roll the dough out on a floured surface to 2cm thick and use a pastry cutter to stamp out 12 scones. Place on a non-stick baking tray and cook for 15–20 minutes.
4 To make the garnish, cut the sun-dried tomatoes into 24. Mix together the yogurt, chives and black pepper to taste.
5 When the corn scones are cooked, remove from the oven and leave to cool. When cool, cut in half and top each half scone with the spiked yogurt and a slice of sun-dried tomato.

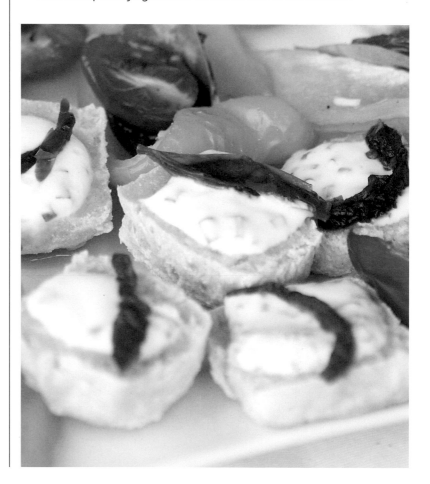

Earl Grey and cherry tea cakes

1 Soak the dried mixed fruit in the hot tea overnight.
2 Preheat the oven to 150C, 300F, gas mark 2. Lightly grease 4 small ovenproof dishes with a little low-fat spread.
3 Place the soaked fruit (and tea) in a mixing bowl. Reserve a few glacé cherries for decoration and add the remainder to the mixing bowl. Add the sugar, flour, egg and mixed spice and mix well. Spoon the mixture into the ovenproof dishes and top with the reserved cherries. Place in the centre of the oven and bake for 45–60 minutes until fully cooked.
4 When cooked, allow to cool in the dishes, then wrap in cellophane and store in an airtight container. To serve cut each tea cake into 4 slices.

SERVES 12
PER SLICE
232 CALORIES
0.9G FAT

SOAKING TIME OVERNIGHT
PREPARATION TIME 10 MINUTES
COOKING TIME 45–60 MINUTES

225g dried mixed fruit
150ml hot Earl Grey tea
100g glacé cherries, chopped
175g dark brown sugar
350g self-raising flour
1 egg, beaten
2 teaspoons mixed spice

TIP *Store the cakes in an airtight container for 2 days to improve the flavour*

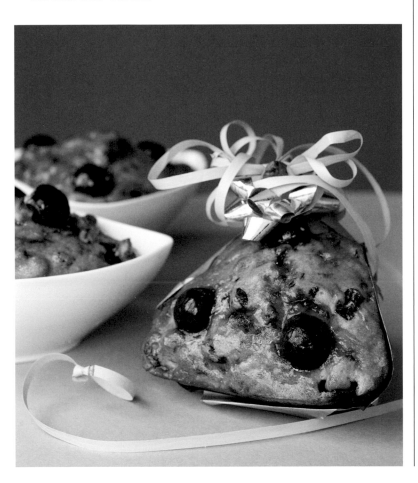

Chocolate yogurt truffles

MAKES 20
PER TRUFFLE
29 CALORIES
1.4G FAT

PREPARATION TIME 10 MINUTES
COOKING TIME 5 MINUTES
SETTING TIME OVERNIGHT

100g dark chocolate (70 %
    cocoa solids)
100g 3 % fat Greek-style
    yogurt
a few drops vanilla essence
cocoa powder to dust

TIP *Wrap the chocolates in cellophane and store in the refrigerator for up a week*

1 Melt the chocolate in a heatproof bowl over a pan of hot water.
2 Allow the chocolate to cool, then slowly stir in the yogurt, taking care not to overmix. Allow to set, ideally overnight.
3 Take small spoonfuls of the mixture and roll between the palms of your hands into little balls. Place on a tray and dust with the cocoa powder.

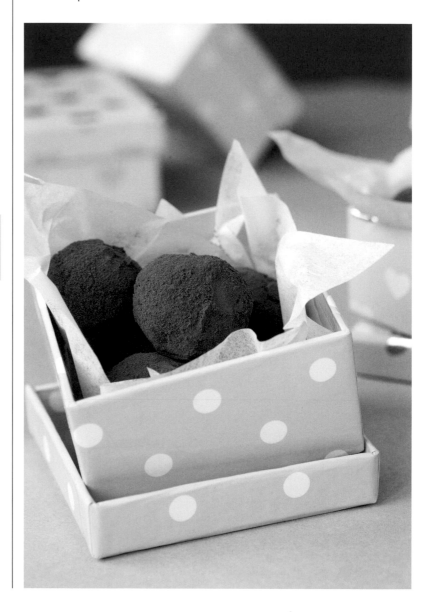

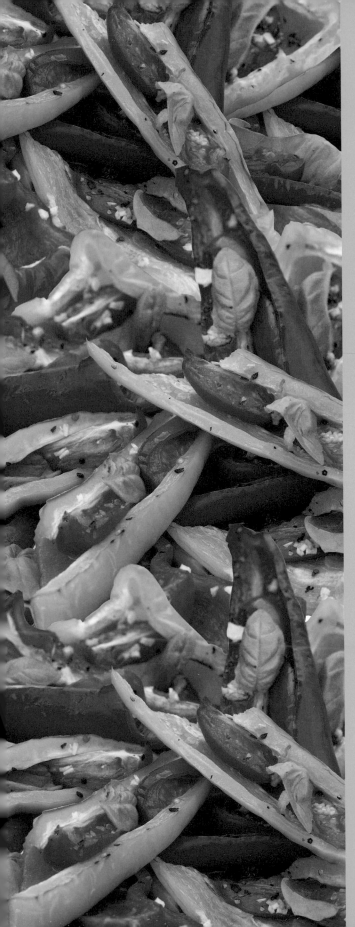

Vegetable side dishes

If you're looking for a new angle on vegetables you'll find some fresh ideas here. Some of these recipes can also be served as vegetarian lunch or dinner options alongside rice, pasta, potatoes or couscous.

Garlic baked tomatoes

SERVES 4
PER SERVING
114 CALORIES
3.8G FAT

PREPARATION TIME 25 MINUTES
COOKING TIME 10–15 MINUTES

4 large beef tomatoes
1 red onion, finely chopped
1 garlic clove, crushed
1 tablespoon chopped fresh
    chives
100g extra light soft cheese
50g low-fat vegetarian
    cheddar-style cheese, grated
1 red pepper, deseeded and
    finely diced
salt and freshly ground black
    pepper

1 Preheat the oven to 200C, 400F, gas mark 6.
2 Wipe the tomatoes with a damp piece of kitchen paper, then slice off the tops and scoop out the seeds with a spoon. Sit the tomatoes in a roasting tray cut-side up.
3 In a small bowl, mix together the onion, garlic, chives, cheese and red pepper, and season with salt and black pepper.
4 Spoon a quarter of the mixture into the centre of each tomato shell. Bake in the oven for 10–15 minutes until cooked through.

TIP *You can turn this into a main meal by serving hot with 1 × 200g oven-baked sweet potato (with skin) per person, vegetables or salad, and sweet chilli sauce*

For added flavour pre-roast the pepper in a hot oven or under a hot grill

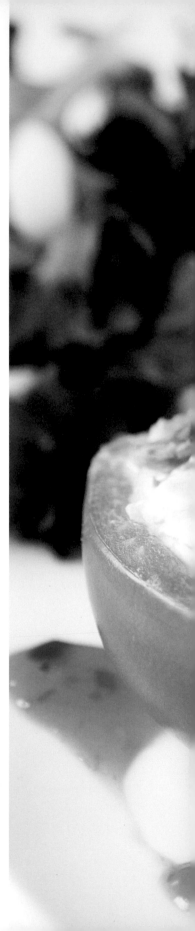

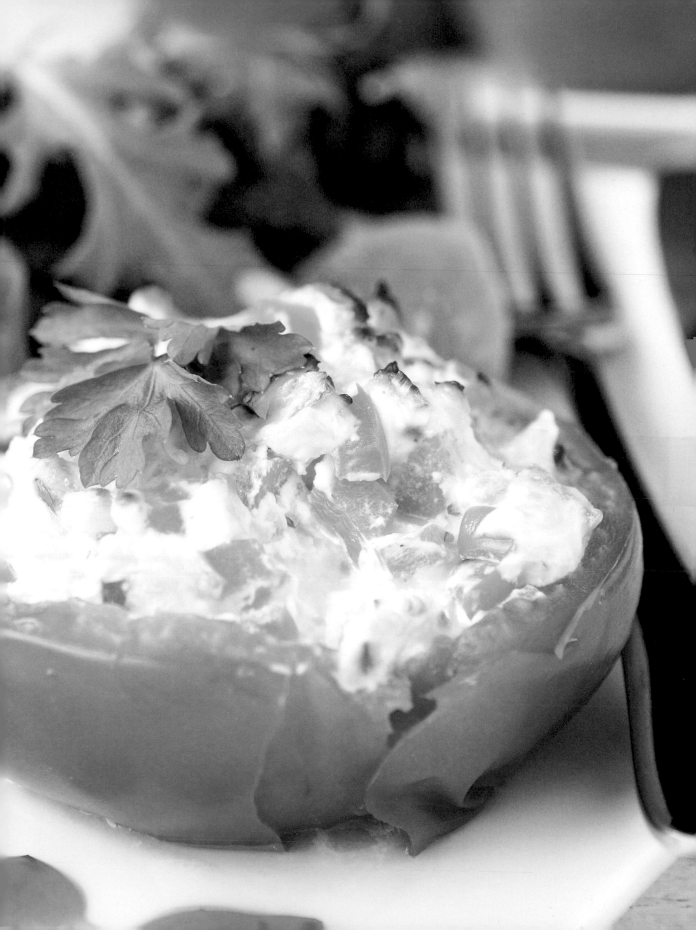

Risotto mushrooms

SERVES 4
PER SERVING
125 CALORIES
0.6G FAT

PREPARATION TIME 10 MINUTES
COOKING TIME 25 MINUTES

4 medium-sized mushrooms
1 garlic clove, crushed
115g Arborio risotto rice
300ml vegetable stock
150ml white wine
2 spring onions, finely chopped
2 tablespoons low-fat fromage
    frais
salt and freshly ground black
    pepper
fresh basil to garnish

1 Preheat the oven to 200C, 400F, gas mark 6.
2 Remove the stalk from the mushrooms. Place the mushrooms
   bottom-side up in a non-stick baking tray and bake in the oven
   for 10 minutes. Remove from the oven and season with salt and
   black pepper.
3 In a non-stick pan, dry-fry the garlic until soft. Add the rice, and
   gradually stir in the stock and wine, allowing the rice to absorb it
   before adding more (this will take between 15 and 20 minutes).
4 Once all the liquid has been added, stir in the chopped spring
   onions. Remove from the heat and fold in the fromage frais.
   Season with salt and freshly ground black pepper to taste.
5 Fill the mushrooms with the rice and garnish with fresh basil.

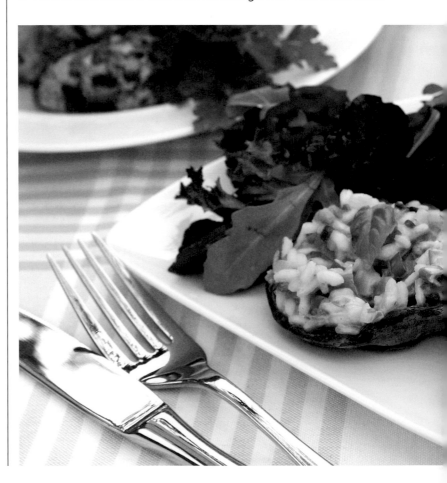

Risotto mushrooms

Courgette and pepper rosti

1 Using the coarse side of a grater, grate the courgettes and red pepper into a mixing bowl. Add the garlic and season with salt and black pepper.
2 Mix in the flour and the beaten egg, along with the parsley.
3 Heat a non-stick frying pan. Spoon 4 separate piles of the mixture into the hot pan, squashing them down with the back of the spoon.
4 Cook over a moderate heat for 5–6 minutes on each side until soft and golden brown.

SERVES 4
PER SERVING
70 CALORIES
2.2G FAT

PREPARATION TIME 10 MINUTES
COOKING TIME 20 MINUTES

225g courgettes
1 red pepper, deseeded
1 garlic clove, crushed
1 tablespoon wholemeal flour
1 egg beaten with 1 tablespoon semi-skimmed milk
1 tablespoon chopped fresh parsley
salt and freshly ground black pepper

TIP *Try these without the garlic as a light breakfast dish*

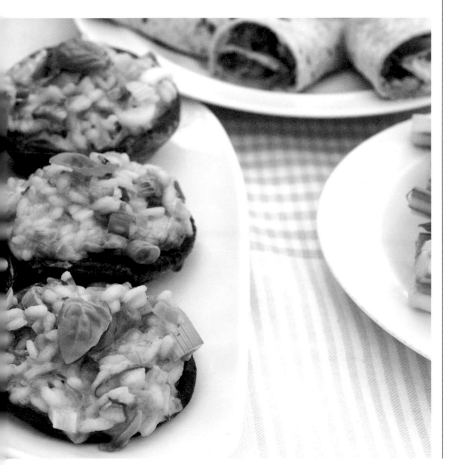

Cheesy baked mushrooms

1 Preheat the oven to 200C, 400F, gas mark 6.
2 Remove the stalks from the mushrooms. Finely chop the stalks and mix with the remaining ingredients except the grated cheese.
3 Spoon the mixture into the mushrooms and top with the grated cheese.
4 Bake in the oven for 15 minutes or until golden brown.

SERVES 4
PER SERVING
66 KCAL
1G FAT

PREPARATION TIME 5 MINUTES
COOKING TIME 15 MINUTES

4 large mushrooms
250g Quark low-fat soft cheese
4 spring onions
1 garlic clove, crushed
1 tablespoon chopped fresh
    herbs
a little fresh lemon zest
20g grated low-fat vegetarian
    cheese
salt and freshly ground black
    pepper to taste

TIP *You can make these mushrooms in advance and keep refrigerated for up to 2 days*

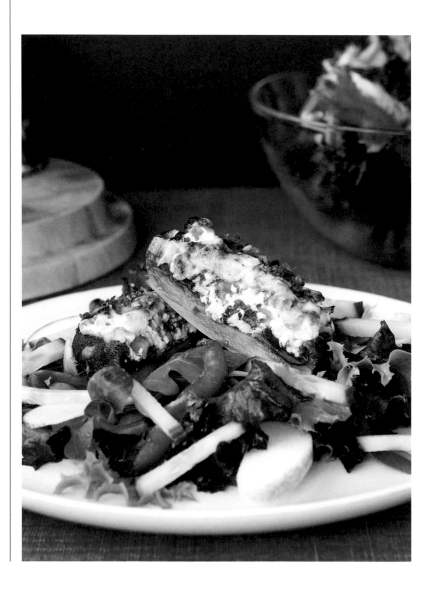

Garlic roast peppers

1 Preheat the oven to 200C, 400F, gas mark 6.
2 Cut the red and yellow peppers into quarters and place in a roasting tray.
3 Cut the tomatoes in half and place a tomato half inside each pepper quarter. Season well with salt and black pepper.
4 Dot small amounts of the chopped garlic inside the peppers.
5 Roast the peppers in the top of the oven for 20–25 minutes until they start to soften. Sprinkle with the chopped basil.

SERVES 4
PER SERVING
27 CALORIES
0.31G FAT

PREPARATION TIME 10 MINUTES
COOKING TIME 15 MINUTES

1 red pepper, deseeded
1 yellow pepper, deseeded
4 cherry tomatoes
1 large garlic clove, finely
    chopped
salt and freshly ground black
    pepper
a few chopped fresh basil leaves
    to garnish

TIP *Use well-ripe tomatoes for a fuller flavour and choose even-sized peppers to ensure they all cook at the same speed*

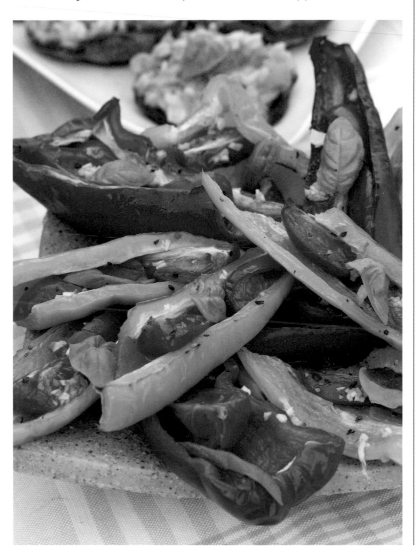

Cumin spiced vegetables

SERVES 4
PER SERVING
93 KCAL
1.3G FAT

PREPARATION TIME 5 MINUTES
COOKING TIME 20 MINUTES

1 red onion, chopped
1 garlic clove, crushed
1 teaspoon cumin seeds
1 teaspoon ground turmeric
300g diced root vegetables
   (swede, carrot, parsnip)
1 teaspoon vegetable stock
   powder
1 small red chilli, sliced
1 red pepper, deseeded and
   diced
1 yellow pepper, deseeded and
   diced
1 × 400g can chopped
   tomatoes
2 tablespoons 3% fat natural
   yogurt
freshly ground black pepper
fresh coriander to serve

TIP *You can also serve with
rice or naan as a meal in itself*

1 Heat a non-stick frying pan, and dry-fry the onion and garlic
   until soft.
2 Add the spices and root vegetables and cook for 1–2 minutes.
   Add the stock powder, chilli, peppers and tomatoes and simmer
   gently for 20 minutes until the vegetables are soft.
3 Just before serving stir in the yogurt.

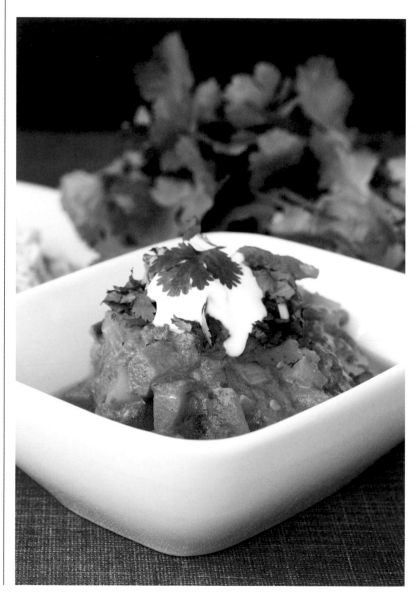

Three colour veg

1 Peel and dice the vegetables. Cook together in a saucepan of boiling water with the vegetable stock cube, then drain and serve.

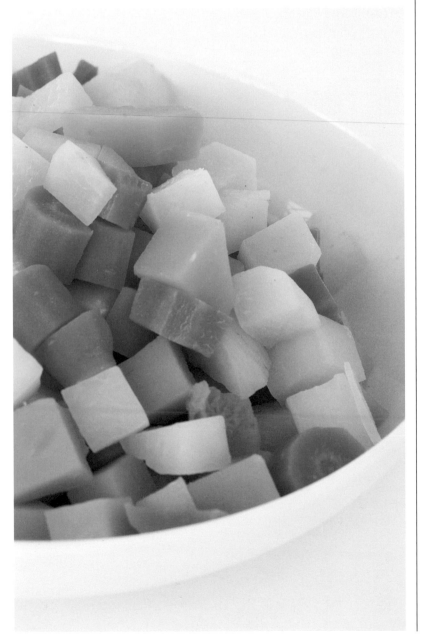

PER 150G SERVING
48 CALORIES
0.4G FAT

PREPARATION TIME 5 MINUTES
COOKING TIME 20 MINUTES

50g butternut squash
50g swede
50g carrots
1 vegetable stock cube

TIP *You can also cook squash on a griddle or barbecue, or bake, split in half and seeds removed, in a non-stick roasting tin placed in a moderate oven for 25–30 minutes*

Spicy sweet potato slices

SERVES 4
PER SERVING
137 CALORIES
1G FAT

PREPARATION TIME 10 MINUTES
COOKING TIME 25–30 MINUTES

4 large sweet potatoes (approx.
    600g total)
1 vegetable stock cube
low-calorie oil spray
2 teaspoons fajita spice mix

1 Preheat the oven to 200C, 400F, gas mark 6.
2 Cut the potatoes into slices and place in a saucepan. Add the stock cube and just cover with water. Bring to the boil and cook for 5 minutes.
3 Drain well and place on a non-stick baking tray. Spray lightly with the oil and then sprinkle the potato slices with the spices on both sides. Place in the oven for 20–25 minutes until golden brown. These go well with grilled steak or gammon.

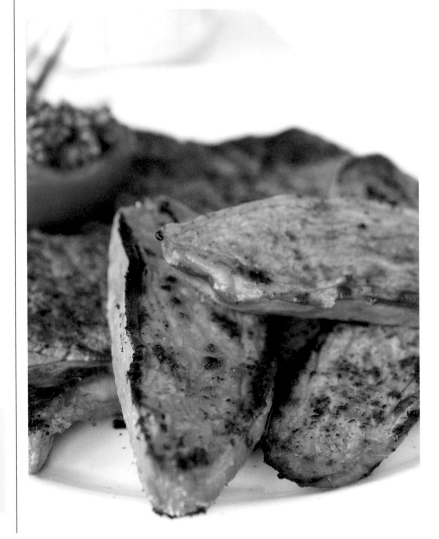

TIP *Fajita spice mix really peps up these potato slices. You can vary the flavour by using other spice mixes and herbs*

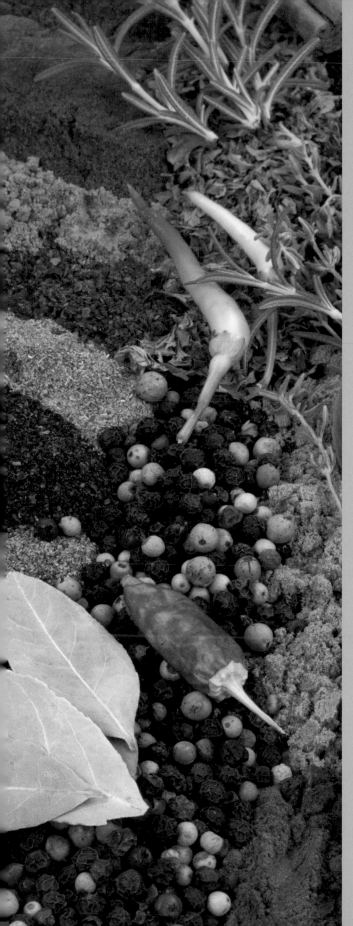

Get saucy

Need to pep up a last-minute dinner party dish, family meal or supper for one? These six simple sauces take only minutes to prepare and you're likely to have all the ingredients to hand in your storecupboard or fridge.

Sweet and sour

SERVES 4
PER SERVING
45 CALORIES
0.01G FAT

1 × 227g can pineapple slices in
   juice
1 tablespoon honey
1 tablespoon tomato purée
1 teaspoon cider vinegar
salt and freshly ground black
   pepper

Serve with: pork, chicken and
   prawns

1 Liquidise the pineapple slices and their juice, and pour into a
   saucepan.
2 Add the honey, tomato purée and cider vinegar. Season with
   salt and black pepper and
   heat through.

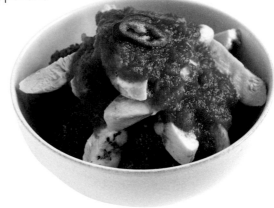

Italian tomato

SERVES 4
PER SERVING
17 CALORIES
0.1G FAT

1 × 400g can tomatoes
1 tablespoon chopped fresh
   mixed herbs
1 garlic clove
salt and freshly ground black
   pepper

Serve with: all meats and grilled
   vegetables

1 Liquidise the tomatoes and their juice, and pour into a
   saucepan.
2 Add the chopped herbs and garlic. Season with salt and black
   pepper and heat through.

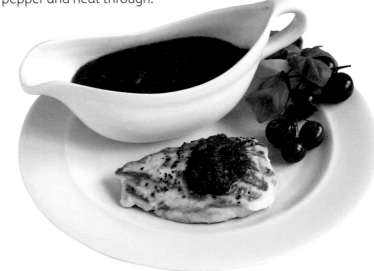

Blackbean express

1 Heat the blackbean sauce, lemon juice and honey in a saucepan and serve.

SERVES 1
PER SERVING
96 CALORIES
0.9G FAT

2 tablespoons blackbean sauce
juice of ½ lemon
1 tablespoon runny honey

Serve with: beef, turkey and
    gammon

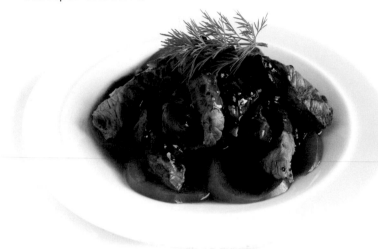

Orange and ginger

1 Heat the orange juice, ginger and honey in a saucepan.
2 Mix the arrowroot with a little cold water and stir into the pan to thicken the sauce, then add the parsley before serving.

SERVES 1
PER SERVING
116 CALORIES
0.09G FAT

juice of 1 orange
1 teaspoon finely chopped fresh
    ginger
1 tablespoon honey
1 teaspoon arrowroot
1 teaspoon chopped fresh
    parsley.

Serve with: white meat and
    vegetables

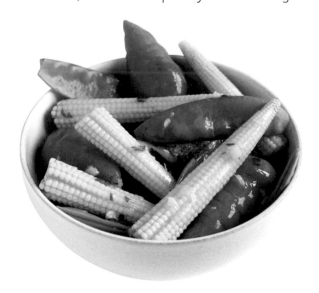

Creamy Thai sauce

SERVES 1
PER SERVING
50 CALORIES
0.3G FAT

2 tablespoons light soy sauce
1 teaspoon lemongrass paste
1 tablespoon tomato purée
300ml water
1 tablespoon virtually fat free
  fromage frais
2 basil leaves, finely shredded

Serve with: fish, beans and all
  meats

1 Place the soy sauce, lemongrass paste and tomato purée in a saucepan. Add the water and bring to the boil to thicken.
2 Remove from the heat and allow to cool slightly before stirring the fromage frais and basil leaves into the sauce.

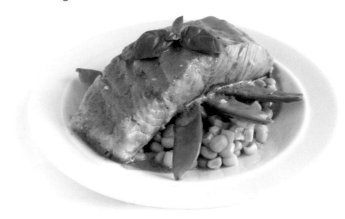

Cheesy mustard sauce

SERVES 4
PER SERVING
122 CALORIES
2.2G FAT

600ml skimmed milk
1 teaspoon vegetable stock
  powder
1 tablespoon cornflour
a little cold milk
1 tablespoon grainy mustard
100g Rosemary Conley mature
  cheese, grated
1 tablespoon finely chopped
  fresh chives

Serve with: fish, ham and
  vegetables

1 In a saucepan, heat the milk with the vegetable stock powder.
2 Slake the cornflour with a little cold milk and whisk into the hot milk, stirring continuously to any prevent lumps forming.
3 Stir in the mustard and grated cheese, and finish with the chives.

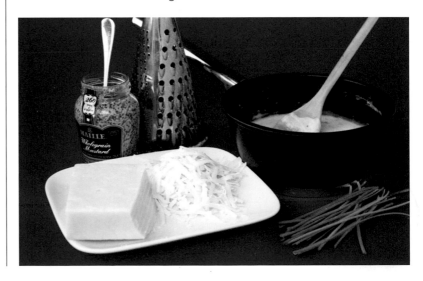

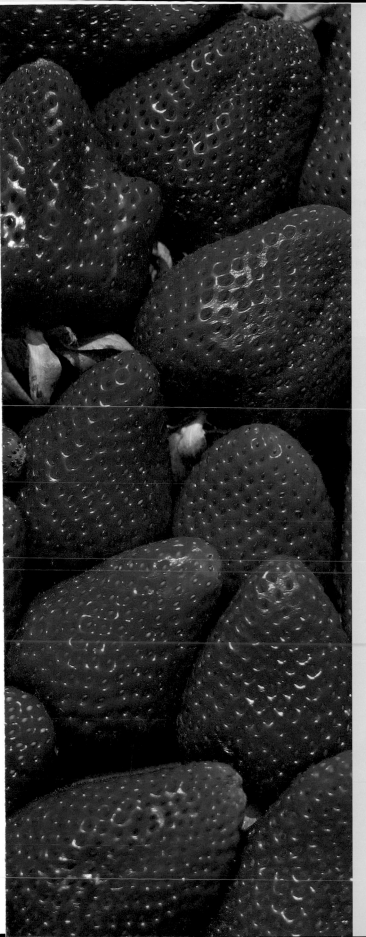

Puddings to please

Even when you're trying to shed a few pounds, puddings don't have to be a no-no. And there's plenty of choice here, from simple, fruit-based concoctions to more elaborate offerings. So take your pick and enjoy!

Sticky chocolate pudding

SERVES 8
PER SERVING
151 KCAL
3.3G FAT

PREPARATION TIME 10 MINUTES
COOKING TIME 30 MINUTES

for the pudding
100g dark brown sugar
100g St Ivel Extra Light
    margarine
2 eggs
25g cocoa
75g plain flour
1 teaspoon baking powder
1 × 100g pot virtually fat free
    fromage frais to serve

for the topping
2 teaspoons cocoa powder
2 teaspoons brown sugar
2 teaspoons boiling water

TIP *Cooking this pudding in a loaf mould makes it easier to cut into slices for serving*

1 Preheat the oven to 150C, 300F, gas mark 2. Lightly grease a loaf mould.
2 Mix together all the pudding ingredients in a bowl, using an electric whisk.
3 Pour the mixture in the prepared loaf mould. Bake in the centre of the oven for 30 minutes until firm to the touch. Remove from the oven.
4 Mix together the topping ingredients and pour over the pudding. Return to the oven for 5 minutes before serving.
5 Serve warm with the fromage frais.

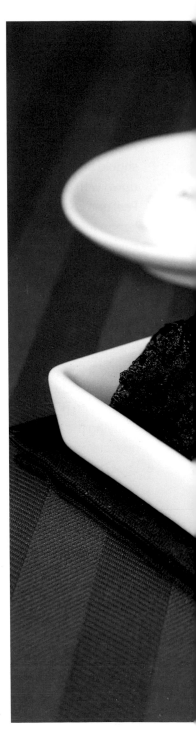

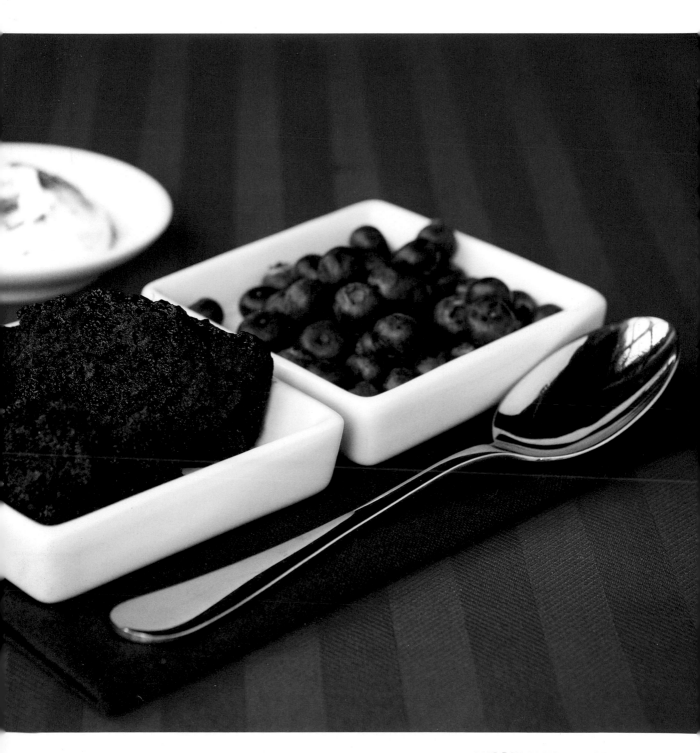

Personal calorie allowance (women)

Check against your current weight and age range to find the ideal daily calorie allowance that will give you a healthy rate of weight loss after you've completed the two-week Fat Attack Fortnight Diet.

Women aged 18–29

Body Weight

Stones	Kilos	Calories
7	45	1147
7.5	48	1194
8	51	1241
8.5	54	1288
9	57	1335
9.5	60.5	1382
10	64	1430
10.5	67	1477
11	70	1524
11.5	73	1571
12	76	1618
12.5	80	1665
13	83	1712
13.5	86	1760
14	89	1807
14.5	92	1854
15	95.5	1901
15.5	99	1948
16	102	1995
16.5	105	2043
17	108	2090
17.5	111	2137
18	115	2184
18.5	118	2231
19	121	2278
19.5	124	2325
20	127	2373

Women aged 30–59

Body Weight

Stones	Kilos	Calories
7	45	1208
7.5	48	1233
8	51	1259
8.5	54	1285
9	57	1311
9.5	60.5	1337
10	64	1373
10.5	67	1389
11	70	1414
11.5	73	1440
12	76	1466
12.5	80	1492
13	83	1518
13.5	86	1544
14	89	1570
14.5	92	1595
15	95.5	1621
15.5	99	1647
16	102	1673
16.5	105	1699
17	108	1725
17.5	111	1751
18	115	1776
18.5	118	1802
19	121	1828
19.5	124	1854
20	127	1880

Women aged 60–74

Body Weight

Stones	Kilos	Calories
7	45	1048
7.5	48	1073
8	51	1099
8.5	54	1125
9	57	1151
9.5	60.5	1176
10	64	1202
10.5	67	1228
11	70	1254
11.5	73	1279
12	76	1305
12.5	80	1331
13	83	1357
13.5	86	1382
14	89	1408
14.5	92	1434
15	95.5	1460
15.5	99	1485
16	102	1511
16.5	105	1537
17	108	1563
17.5	111	1588
18	115	1614
18.5	118	1640
19	121	1666
19.5	124	1691
20	127	1717

Personal calorie allowance (men)

Check against your current weight and age range to find the ideal daily calorie allowance that will give you a healthy rate of weight loss after you've completed the two-week Fat Attack Fortnight Diet.

Men aged 18–29			Men aged 30–59			Men aged 60–74		
Body Weight			Body Weight			Body Weight		
Stones	Kilos	Calories	Stones	Kilos	Calories	Stones	Kilos	Calories
7	45	1363	7	45	1384	7	45	1232
7.5	48	1411	7.5	48	1421	7.5	48	1270
8	51	1459	8	51	1457	8	51	1307
8.5	54	1507	8.5	54	1494	8.5	54	1345
9	57	1555	9	57	1530	9	57	1383
9.5	60.5	1602	9.5	60.5	1567	9.5	60.5	1421
10	64	1650	10	64	1603	10	64	1459
10.5	67	1698	10.5	67	1640	10.5	67	1497
11	70	1746	11	70	1676	11	70	1535
11.5	73	1794	11.5	73	1713	11.5	73	1573
12	76	1842	12	76	1749	12	76	1611
12.5	80	1890	12.5	80	1786	12.5	80	1649
13	83	1938	13	83	1822	13	83	1687
13.5	86	1986	13.5	86	1859	13.5	86	1725
14	89	2034	14	89	1895	14	89	1763
14.5	92	2082	14.5	92	1932	14.5	92	1801
15	95.5	2129	15	95.5	1968	15	95.5	1839
15.5	99	2177	15.5	99	2005	15.5	99	1877
16	102	2225	16	102	2041	16	102	1915
16.5	105	2273	16.5	105	2078	16.5	105	1953
17	108	2321	17	108	2114	17	108	1991
17.5	111	2369	17.5	111	2151	17.5	111	2028
18	115	2417	18	115	2187	18	115	2066
18.5	118	2465	18.5	118	2224	18.5	118	2104
19	121	2513	19	121	2260	19	121	2142
19.5	124	2561	19.5	124	2297	19.5	124	2180
20	127	2609	20	127	2333	20	127	2218

Weight-loss progress chart

	weight now	pounds/kg lost	total loss to date
Start day date:			
Week 1 date:			
Week 2 date:			
Week 3 date:			
Week 4 date:			
Week 5 date:			
Week 6 date:			
Week 7 date:			
Week 8 date:			
Week 9 date:			
Week 10 date:			
Week 11 date:			
Week 12 date:			
Week 13 date:			

Weight-loss graph

Plot your weight-loss progress on the grid each week from 'START HERE'. Your graph should show a line from 'START HERE' descending towards the bottom right side of the chart.

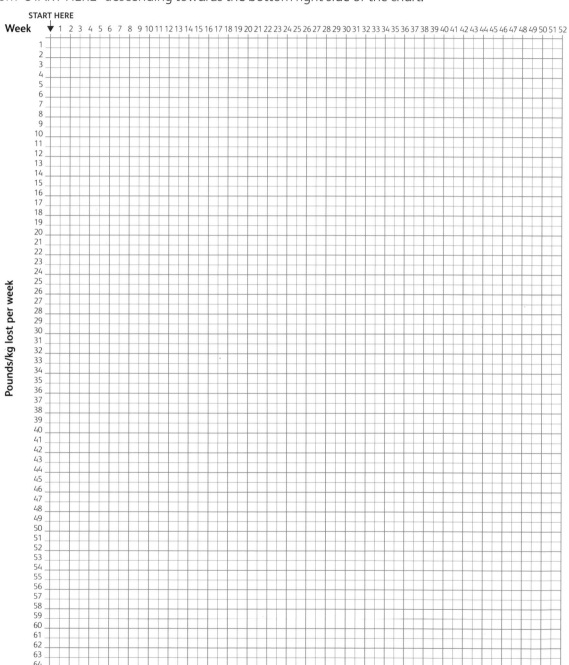

Inch-loss chart

date	weight	bust	waist	hips

widest part	top of thighs left	right	above knees left	right	upper arms left	right

BW 1/11